Beyond Menopause: Your Playbook for Strength, Vitality and Purpose in Midlife

Table of Content

Introduction

Menopause can feel like an ending. Your periods stop, signaling your fertility has declined along with key hormones like estrogen. Hot flashes, trouble sleeping, weight gain, and other unwelcome physical and emotional changes may have you wondering if your vitality has peaked. News headlines only amplify the gloom and doom, warning about increased health risks in midlife for everything from heart disease to dementia. No wonder many women approach menopause with trepidation or dread.

But this transition does not have to signify decline or mark the beginning of the end. Far from it! While menopause heralds the close of your reproductive years, it opens the door to an entire second act filled with freedom, wisdom, meaning, and joy. The key is tuning into and caring for your body's changing needs while expanding the possibilities for purpose and passion. *Beyond Menopause: Your Playbook for Strength, Vitality, and Purpose In Midlife* provides science-backed strategies and empowering mindset shifts to help you do just that.

Why a Playbook?

Just like world-class athletes gear up for the next championship game with a winning playbook full of proven strategies from nutrition to recovery, you need a plan to optimize your performance and wellbeing during the menopausal transition and beyond. Consider this book your coaching guide. In the first half, we'll dig into the physiological changes of menopause and equip you with concrete solutions to manage symptoms, maintain health, and adapt your fitness approach. In the second half, we'll game out thriving in relationships, pursuing revitalizing goals around purpose, passion, sensuality and more.

You'll find sample workouts, nutrition advice, stress busters, relationship builders, passion projects, financial plans and other tactical tools. But beyond the nitty gritty what-to-eat-and-do advice lies a more profound opportunity...

From Surviving to Thriving

Instead of just coping with menopause, you can harness this transition to craft your best life yet. Beyond managing symptoms, you can leverage hormonal changes to transform how you fuel, train, work, love, parent, contribute and more. Emerging science confirms women can achieve awe-inspiring fitness at any age while reducing risks for nearly all major diseases through smart lifestyle strategies. And freed from biological fertility or full-time parenting duties, postmenopausal women often direct energy towards rewarding goals that amplify purpose, community impact and fulfillment.

Own Your Transition, Own Your Power

Menopause has gotten a bad rap in western cultures, portrayed as an awkward inconvenience, something broken that increases vulnerability. But the truth universally rings that with age comes power, wisdom and expanded capability built from experience. Menopause marks not the beginning of decline but your next ascent!

The key is recognizing and mastering the changes in your body, relationships and world rather than resisting them. *Beyond Menopause* puts you back in the driver's seat of your health and life. You'll walk away from this book with inspiration from those thriving through menopause, science-backed recommendations customized to your unique needs, and a personalized playbook to elevate your vitality, performance, sensuality and purpose over the next 30+ years. Think of menopause not as stepping back but leaping ahead. Your vibrant future filled with strength, intimacy, meaning and joy awaits! Let's get started.

Part I: Understanding Your Changing Body

Before strategizing how to optimize your health, fitness and vibe through menopause, you need to understand what's happening inside your body. Consider Part I your physiology primer for the changes ahead.

Here we'll dig into:

- What menopause really means and the hormonal shifts behind your symptoms

- How estrogen, progesterone, testosterone and other key players change as your ovaries gradually retire from regular egg production

- The effects of these hormonal fluctuations on your sleep, weight, energy, moods, health risks and fitness potential

- How perimenopause, menopause stages and timelines affect women differently

Understanding the science equips you to work *with* your transition not fight against it. You'll discover how to leverage natural shifts to enhance wellness or gracefully adapt to what you can't control. Think how world-class athletes master essential bio-mechanics to optimize training and avoid injury. Similarly, learning your hormonal patterns allows customizing lifestyle, fitness and nutrition to your phase.

Yet menopausal physiology remains shrouded in mystery, misinformation and taboo. Few women realize the breadth of influence declining estrogen and progesterone have on health and performance or understand the opportunities past peak fertility. My goal is to change that through simple, empowering science that breeds action.

Use Part I to identify changes you may be experiencing now or soon. Discover how menopause intersects with chronic conditions you already manage. Most importantly, walk away realizing the breadth of what you *can* proactively do to feel great in your body as hormones shift. Too many women still perceive menopause management as limited to treating hot flashes, when nothing could be further from the truth!

Understanding exactly how your changing physiology impacts fitness, fueling, health risks and flow states provides a foundation for smarter solutions. Use the science in Part I to build motivation, destroy myths and craft a custom playbook for your transition. Thriving through menopause begins with knowledge, listening to your body's signals and translating that wisdom into better self-care. Turn the page to start your education!

The Physiology of Menopause

Let's start at the beginning by defining menopause and unpacking exactly what causes all those fun symptoms like hot flashes.

Menopause: What Does It Mean?

Menopause simply marks the end of menstrual periods signaling your ovaries have stopped releasing eggs. It's a normal biological transition all women experience, usually between the ages of 45-55.

The hallmark of menopause is when you haven't had a period for 12 full months. That point in time is called natural menopause. The average age for the final period hovers around 51 but onset varies widely. Menopause generally occurs earlier for smokers or women with chronic health issues.

Perimenopause, the transition years leading up to this one year mark, is actually the rockiest hormonal phase that causes most disruptive symptoms. This winding down of fertility and menstruation can start up to 10 years beforehand. Some women barely notice perimenopause changes while others feel blindsided by unwelcome shifts.

Rather than an event, treat menopause as a gradual biological process that unfolds over years or even decades. Hormone levels fluctuate but decline progressively until eventually ovaries shut down egg production entirely. Declining ovarian function means your ovaries make less of the sex hormones estrogen and progesterone. Lower estrogen is the main driver of menopause related changes, but it affects every woman differently.

What Causes Menopause?

You're born with around 1-2 million eggs in your ovaries and lose thousands per month until your egg supply becomes too low to keep a regular menstrual cycle going. This declining egg supply correlates directly with lowering estrogen and progesterone.

Your pituitary gland and hypothalamus control ovarian function and sex hormone production through an intricate dance of feedback loops. As your ovaries become less responsive, these master control glands essentially crank up production of follicle stimulating hormone (FSH) and luteinizing hormone (LH) to whip your ovaries into action. This overcompensation is why FSH and LH levels skyrocket through perimenopause and menopause even as estrogen drops.

Here's a simple way to remember the gist: Your brain shouts instructions to produce more estrogen and release eggs ---> Your ovaries say "Nah I'm good!" and keep losing eggs/making less estrogen ---> Your brain freaks out and screams louder at your stubborn ovaries ---> The pattern continues until ovaries totally tap out.

This communication breakdown means your reproductive hormone balance unravels. The good news? Understanding what's behind your symptoms allows optimizing lifestyle for your situation.

Now let's explore exactly how declining sex hormones impact the rest of your body beyond simply ending periods.

How Does Menopause Impact You Beyond Fertility?

The effects of lowering estrogen and progesterone span far beyond your reproductive health. Every cell in your body has receptors for these hormones so changes reverberate widely. Here's an overview of some key impacts:

Metabolic Effects

Lower estrogen is closely linked to increased belly fat storage and insulin resistance. This makes managing blood sugar levels and weight gain extra challenging through menopause, even if diet stays consistent. Declining estrogen also negatively impacts cholesterol ratios. Together these metabolic shifts increase risk for diabetes, heart disease and stroke. We tackle solutions in nutrition and exercise chapters.

Bone Loss

Estrogen plays a key role building bone density during young adulthood to peak around age 30. As estrogen drops, bone breakdown accelerates leading to rapid loss of bone mineral density for several years. If unchecked, this osteopenia leads to full blown osteoporosis and greater fracture risks. Get ahead of bone loss through weight training, nutrition and monitoring.

Hot Flashes & Night Sweats

The exact mechanism remains unknown but research links hot flashes to changing estrogen communicating with your hypothalamus, the body's temperature regulation center. Low estrogen levels cause it to become hypersensitive leading to rapid dilating of blood vessels and flushing. Progesterone withdrawal likely also plays a role. Not all women experience hot flashes, but 75% do to some degree.

Vaginal Atrophy

Declining estrogen thins vaginal walls leading to dryness, irritation, inflammation and increased infections. Discomfort and pain during sex results along with more frequent UTIs or yeast infections. Over the counter lubricants and moisturizers can ease symptoms.

Breast Changes

Density and tissue composition shifts due to lower progesterone levels and milk producing glands shrinking after childbearing years. Tenderness, fullness or pain are common. Lower estrogen increases breast cancer risk slightly.

Emotional Changes

Estrogen, progesterone, serotonin and other hormone pathways closely impact mood regulation and brain health. Some women experience anxiety, depression, trouble focusing, memory lapses or emotional sensitivity during the menopausal transition years. Coping with unwelcome physical changes certainly contributes to feeling irritated as well!

Sleep Disruption

From night sweats to frequent waking, sleep suffers for up to 60% of perimenopausal and menopausal women. Yet inadequate sleep intensifies other symptoms like low energy, trouble focusing, weight gain and emotional volatility. Supporting restful sleep is key.

Skin, Hair & Nails

Collagen production slows while skin becomes thinner and drier leading to wrinkles and crepiness. Stubborn fat accumulation plus muscle loss from aging can exacerbate sagging. Many women also notice their hair seems to thin with more scalp visible or nails become more brittle.

This snapshot just touches the surface of estrogen's wide ranging impacts that intensify the menopausal transition rollercoaster. Keep reading for concrete solutions to smooth out your ride. Forearmed with physiological knowledge, you can customize tactics to alleviate unwanted effects and set yourself up for health and vitality in coming decades.

Now that we've covered the key mechanisms and effects of menopause, let's explore how this winding down progresses in phases. Understanding timing equips you to anticipate changes down the line.

Stages of Menopausal Transition

Perimenopause, menopause, and postmenopause each have distinct hormonal profiles that unfold over years. Some women sail through the flux in hormone levels with barely a blip. Others struggle feeling like they drew the short stick as their bodies change rapidly. When and how dramatically estrogen declines determines symptoms. Let's break down the stages:

Perimenopause

Defined as the 5-10 years leading up to your final period, perimenopause onset happens gradually making early signs easy to overlook or attribute to other causes like aging, life stress, or poor health habits. Changes emerge slowly then eventually speed up as you near your final period.

During perimenopause estrogen levels fluctuate significantly - often wildly veering up and down day to day. You might feel great one week then hit a wall of exhaustion, mood crashes and other symptoms the next. Extended cycles with long or erratic time gaps between periods result along with lighter, shorter or heavy bleeding at odd times.

Symptoms like hot flashes, night sweats, trouble focusing, poor sleep, low libido, and vaginal dryness start for some women during early stage perimenopause. Weight gain and insulin resistance can also intensify years before your final period.

Menopause

By definition you've reached menopause 12 months after your last menstrual cycle finishes. Maximum estrogen drop occurs during the year surrounding your final period when most severe symptoms like hot flashes and night sweats peak for women who experience them.

Postmenopause (up to 5 years past final period) still entails major hormone adjustments as your ovaries continue producing less estrogen along with progesterone and testosterone. Symptoms often continue similar intensity for a year or more before gradually easing. Many women use short term hormone therapy during this unstable time for symptom relief.

Postmenopause

A decade or more past your last period, most women notice life settling into a calmer, more predictable pattern as hormones stabilize at lower levels. However metabolism and other effects of estrogen deficiency persist along with risks like heart disease and osteoporosis. Committing long term to protective lifestyle strategies pays dividends now.

Remember menopause unfolds gradually over years - even decades - not overnight. Be patient with your body amidst temporary chaos knowing that this too shall pass! Take comfort that for 80% of women the most disruptive symptoms resolve within five years of that final period.

Now let's move onto clarifying other key language about induced menopause, early menopause, hormone therapy and more.

Clearing Up Menopause Terminology Confusion

Here's a quick guide to other menopause related terms and topics that cause lots of confusion:

- *Early or premature menopause* refers to women who stop menstruating before age 40 either naturally or from medical interventions like hysterectomy. This puts them at greater long term health risks from years more estrogen deficiency.

- *Surgical menopause* means menstruation halts suddenly rather than gradually because of medical interventions like ovary removal or hysterectomy. Hormone changes happen abruptly compared to natural winding down with menopause.

- *Induced menopause* describes menstruation stopping due to chemotherapy, radiation, medications or other treatments usually for serious medical conditions.

- *Postmenopausal hormone therapy (HT)* involves taking prescription estrogen or progesterone to alleviate moderate to severe symptoms either locally through creams or systemically with oral pills, patches, shots or pellet implants. It remains controversial and entails balancing benefits against health risks like stroke, blood clots and cancer.

- *Bioidentical hormones* refer to manmade hormone therapy compounds with the exact same molecular structure as endogenous estrogen, progesterone and testosterone. They aim to be identical to your natural hormones but research about risks and efficacy remains ongoing.

- *Compounded hormones* means a pharmacy specially prepares customized doses and combinations of hormones in creams, gels or pellet implants based on your needs. Quality control and purity vary widely between compounding pharmacies.

Hopefully this physiology primer paves the way for you to understand the coming chapters outlining specific solutions to manage symptoms, maintain glowing health and thrive during the menopausal transition and beyond! Our bodies change but self care skills and knowledge remain our best allies.

Common Symptoms and Health Effects

Now that you understand the physiology behind what causes periods to stop during the menopausal transition, let's cover specifics on the most common symptoms along with related health conditions.

Remember, every woman experiences fluctuating and declining hormones differently based on genetics, lifestyle and health status. You may breeze through peri-menopause feeling fabulous while your best friend struggles with disruptive symptoms. Knowledge is power when it comes to managing changes though!

This chapter outlines the breadth of possible effects in the key areas of:

- Hot Flashes, Night Sweats & More
- Weight Gain & Body Composition Changes
- Energy Levels, Moods & Cognitive Function
- Sleep Disruption
- Sexual Health Effects
- Other Common Symptoms

Armed with insight, you can determine which apply to you and laser focus solutions there versus wasting effort on issues you don't struggle with. Let's start with the infamous hot flash!

Hot Flashes, Night Sweats & More

Sporadic heat waves resulting in flushed, sweaty skin along with an elevated heart rate define hot flashes and their nighttime counterparts - night sweats. Most women do experience them to some degree. They stem from decreasing estrogen interacting with your temperature regulation center leading blood vessels near skin to rapidly dilate and then cool again quickly. Triggers range from stress to warm rooms to spicy foods. Here's what to know:

- **Timing & Duration** – Hot flashes often start in perimenopause and peak in the year after your final period when estrogen levels are lowest then become less frequent over 2-5 years. In 10% of women they persist long term or start after menopause is established. Night sweats in particular disrupt sleep quality during this time.

- **Severity** – Frequency ranges from occasional mild flushing to severe sweating that empties bladders or soaks clothes/sheets daily. Pay attention to aggravating lifestyle triggers you can mitigate.

- **Management Tips** – Document your personal patterns around timing, length, severity and triggers. This allows customizing solutions like layering clothing, using fans/AC strategically, avoiding triggers, practicing relaxation skills or taking menopausal supplements.

Beyond merely feeling overheated, let's cover other common symptoms related to declining hormones.

Weight Gain & Body Composition

Up to 90% of women gain unwanted weight and extra body fat during perimenopause and menopause – typically between 10-15 lbs long term. Unfortunately excess fat often deposits around your midsection contributing to increased risks of high blood pressure, cholesterol abnormalities, cardiovascular disease, diabetes and stroke. Why? Beyond slowing metabolism, dropping estrogen directly promotes insulin resistance which makes you more prone to storing belly fat and blood sugar dysregulation. Compounding factors include aging muscle loss, medication use, poor sleep and low energy for activity.

Pay close attention during perimenopause not just menopause. Weight often creeps up gradually at first over years making it hard to pinpoint hormone changes as the cause. Don't accept weight gain as inevitable! The nutrition and fitness chapters will cover specific strategies reversing estrogen-related factors leading to middle aged weight gain. Taking control now improves not just looks but lifelong disease risk.

Energy, Moods & Cognitive Changes

Up to 80% of menopausal women report issues like fatigue, irritability, anxiety or depression and "brain fog" with memory or concentration lapses when estrogen declines. The reasons stem from many factors:

- Hot flashes and night sweats depleting sleep

- Blood sugar swings and inflammation

- Thyroid issues exacerbating low energy

- Medications plus supplements decreasing mental sharpness

- Stress, grief, life changes or trauma

- Physical discomfort from symptoms like joint pain or bladder issues

Mood disorders and cognition challenges often overlap. Feeling blah saps motivation causing you to skip workouts, overeat comfort foods, skimp on self care and sink into a negative cycle. Or painful sex and vaginal dryness strain intimacy in relationships amplifying emotional volatility and mental chatter.

Lifestyle strategies like better sleep, stress management and exercise pay dividends for perking up both energy and outlook. Understanding the physiological drivers means you aren't imagining troubles or solely responsible for "fixing your mood". Have patience with the process and lean on support.

Sleep Disruption

Insomnia and poor sleep plague up to 60% of menopausal women often starting in perimenopause before other symptoms manifest strongly. Declining progesterone directly plays a role, but culprits also include night sweats, anxiety, bladder issues and even painful joints or muscles that prohibit restful sleep. Top consequences encompass low energy, trouble focusing, emotional reactivity and overeating or cravings. Prioritizing healthy sleep and self-care makes every other aspect of menopause transition easier!

Document your own sleep patterns for insight. Do you have trouble falling asleep? Wake frequently? Experience vivid dreams or night sweats? Kick off covers from hot flashes then get chilled? Understanding your issues allows targeted solutions like cooling techniques, herbal supplements, pillows between knees for joint relief or cognitive behavioral therapy for insomnia.

Sexual Health Effects

From vaginal dryness and shrinking tissue elasticity to problems orgasming or plummeting testosterone impacting libido, sexual health suffers for many women at menopause. Up to half experience painful intercourse, burning or irritation. Beyond physical reasons, body image fears, stressors, relationship discord or medication side effects also often tank sex drive and satisfaction. Don't assume issues in the bedroom mean intimacy has to decline!

Know solutions exist from lubricants and moisturizers to pelvic floor therapy, couples counseling and mindset shifts. Explore hormone balancing medications if needed too. While no woman escapes aging, nurturing intimacy and sensuality can still blossom in this season. Expect evolution in what arouses you, how your body responds and ways to nurture relationships.

Other Common Symptoms

Let's quickly cover remaining issues tied to shifting estrogen, progesterone and testosterone:

- **Urinary incontinence or urgency** from thinner urethral tissues along with risk for recurrent UTIs

- **Joint pain and muscle aches** as collagen production declines reducing flexibility

- N **erve pain, numbness or tingling** from tissue drying and thinning

- I **ncreased dental problems** like gingivitis as bone loss includes mouth and jaw

- **Hair, skin and nail changes** like thinning hair, wrinkling or brittle nails

- **Gastrointestinal issues** like constipation from slower transit times

- **Headaches** and migraines

- **Breast pain or swelling**

Review common symptoms knowing most resolve in the years following menopause as your body chemistry stabilizes. Some clearly prompt early action like addressing bone loss or heart disease risks. For issues like hot flashes focus on relief until they pass. Either way, you've got this!

Now let's examine increased risks for major health conditions along with prevention opportunities. Knowledge is power when it comes to reducing disease vulnerability in the decades beyond menopause.

Increased Health Risks & Protective Strategies

While menopause itself doesn't cause illness or chronic diseases directly, losing estrogen long term correlated to significantly higher incidence of the following conditions:

- Cardiovascular disease

- Osteoporosis

- Diabetes & metabolic syndrome

- Certain cancers

- Alzheimer's disease

- Autoimmune conditions

- Liver disease

- Eye & dental diseases

The magnitude of increased relative risks spans from 25% higher for heart disease or stroke up to 300% greater chance of vaginal atrophy or dry eye disease for postmenopausal women compared young adults. Sounds scary doesn't it!

Here's the good news - adopting healthy lifestyle habits effectively minimizes heightened vulnerability for ALL major diseases after menopause despite hormone changes being out of your control. Science confirms women can largely eliminate risks through reasonable nutrition, activity, sleep and stress management steps according to numerous recent studies.

Let's examine key health concerns in more detail along with proactive solutions:

Heart Health After Menopause

Cardiovascular disease remains the #1 killer of women as estrogen drops after midlife. Cholesterol ratios shift to more artery damaging LDL particles, triglycerides rise, and other metabolic changes like insulin resistance or abdominal weight gain exacerbate inflammation and blood vessel damage. Another key reason stems from endothelium - the delicate inner skin of arteries - becoming more prone to plaques and lesions without estrogen helping facilitate nitric oxide benefits that keep vessels flexible.

Your action plan for prevention leans heavily on adopting heart healthy nutrition and lifestyle habits before menopause onset:

- Engage aerobic activity 30+ minutes daily

- Strength train 2-3x/week

- Eat anti-inflammatory whole foods

- Monitor blood sugar, triglycerides and cholesterol

- Discuss statins or prescription estrogen with your doctor if at high risk

Bone Loss Protection Strategies

Osteopenia and osteoporosis result from estrogen declining to help regulate bone building cell activity in your youth. This leads to gradual bone mineral density loss and vulnerability to fractures. Women lose up to 20% of bone mass in the 5 to 7 years following menopause, making early screening and prevention tactics essential.

Recommendations for preserving bone health include:

- Get baseline DEXA scan at perimenopause onset

- Consume plenty calcium rich foods

- Take 1000-2000 IU vitamin D3 daily

- Incorporate weight bearing and resistance exercise

- If needed add bisphosphonates, hormone therapy, etc under medical care

Diabetes & Metabolic Disease Risks

As mentioned previously, diminished estrogen closely associates with increased visceral belly fat, poor blood sugar regulation and insulin resistance - all paving the way for type 2 diabetes and metabolic disorders. Women with diabetes demonstrate more severe menopause symptoms too. In addition to diabetes posing its own health threats, having chronically high blood sugar and lipids accelerates development of heart and neurodegenerative diseases.

Guard against metabolic disease risks by:

- Achieving or maintaining healthy body composition

- Choosing whole, fiber rich complex carbs

- Monitoring fasting blood glucose and HbA1c

- Taking medications or incorporating functional supplements as directed by your doctor.

Cancer Risks After Menopause

Breast and reproductive organ cancers no longer intensify after menopause, but risks for others including lung, colorectal, pancreatic and skin cancers climb exponentially compared to younger adults. Interestingly multiple studies found smoking, excess body fat, poor diet quality and not exercising essentially eliminated extra cancer risks in postmenopausal women and older adults.

Your action plan for cancer defense includes:

- Eating anti-inflammatory whole foods

- Engaging moderate activity daily

- Protecting skin from excessive sun exposure

- Getting regular age - and risk- appropriate cancer screenings

In Conclusion

While menopause transitions bring unique symptoms and evolving health considerations, you now understand the breadth of proven solutions within your control. Through personalized lifestyle tweaks, community support and preventative medical care, you can alleviate discomforts, shrink long term disease threats and continue thriving in mind, body and spirit more decades.

Hopefully this overview of common symptoms, related conditions and protective strategies allows you to pinpoint current struggles and map out priorities for feeling your best in coming years.

Impacts on Your Fitness & Performance

By now you've realized the breadth of changes underway during the menopausal transition spanning energy, metabolism, body composition, sleep, cognition and more. Let's dig into specifics on how declining estrogen and these widespread shifts affect your fitness, athletic performance and active lifestyle.

The interplay between hormones and training proves complex. Physical movement potently protects health yet adapting activity to match your body's changes remains key as estrogen wanes. Just like an elite athlete wouldn't gut through injuries or overtrain when fatigued, you shouldn't push through joint pain or exhaustion assuming symptoms will just resolve on their own over time.

This chapter covers key impacts on fitness and athletic performance including:

- Musculoskeletal Issues Affecting Movement

- Cardiorespiratory Impacts

- Weight Gain & Body Composition

- Motivation & Mindset Hurdles

Plus how to modify workouts, recovery approaches, and nutrition support during the menopausal transition without losing ground. Let's start with the physical.

Musculoskeletal Changes

Progressive loss of muscle mass, strength and power accelerates during peri-menopause and the years immediately following due to metabolic shifts. Up to 3% loss per year results driven by declining estrogen and testosterone interacting with protein synthesis and neuromuscular pathways.

This steady wasting away of muscle mass fuels faster fat gain and slower resting metabolism. You gradually lose that badass calorie burning engine built through years of training! Additionally collagen production slows, leading to stiffer tendons, ligaments and less flexible joints plus lower bone mineral density.

Together these musculoskeletal effects contribute to feeling creaky and injury prone:

- Joint pain

- Muscle or bone injuries

- Poor mobility, balance and coordination

- Reduced strength and endurance

Without strategically addressing new vulnerabilities through smart training modifications, many women struggle with lackluster race times, strength gains stalling out and feeling discouraged in the gym or on trails.

Pay attention to emerging issues like hip bursitis flare ups, plantar fasciitis or sudden shoulder instability. Your connective tissues and joints now demonstrate less resilience and need additional care against overuse or strain. Luckily both nutrition and training interventions make a world of difference preventing accelerated physical decline during menopause.

Heart, Lung & Endurance Changes

Beyond musculoskeletal discomforts, your cardiorespiratory system feels the effects of menopause too. Maximum oxygen uptake and lactate thresholds crucial for endurance adapt to the declining estrogen party happening inside your body.

Research confirms VO_2 max and heart rates at given paces inevitably drop about 5 to 10% between ages 35 and 60 even in highly trained athletes who keep training methodology constant. For most active women, that decline manifests through feeling more sluggish, winded, or lacking "pop" at usual paces. Race times for similar perceived effort creep slower.

Making matters more complicated, low iron stores or anemia intensify fatigue and oxygen delivering capacity declines too for some women during heavy menstrual bleeding phases earlier in the transition.

Don't automatically assume fading endurance means your best days fell behind you already! Strategic training adjustments to match your changing fitness levels prevent frustration. More on that soon.

Weight Gain & Body Composition

We've covered the perfect metabolic storm caused by declining estrogen and associated insulin resistance, progressive muscle loss, lifestyle stressors and fatigue diminishing activity levels. Simply put - challenged hormone regulation makes gaining fat around the midsection much easier while losing extra padding feels nearly impossible. Even maintaining prior weight now requires extra diligence with food planning and training stimulus.

Excess body fat worsens health risks and makes keeping up fitness levels harder both physically and motivationally. It becomes a self-sabotaging cycle too easy to spiral down as mensural irregularities throw off nutrition habits and workouts.

Commit now not to write off strength training, peloton classes or whatever activities you enjoy. Scale back intensity if needed through this transitional phase rather than quitting completely. Even movement at lower efforts pays worthwhile dividends until you regain momentum. Every step counts when it comes to supporting better body composition, metabolic health and retaining lean mass through menopause.

Motivation & Mindset Pitfalls

Finally, let's address the inner game of menopausal fitness. Declining athletic performance combined with unwelcome body composition changes often trigger motivation nosedives. Negative self-talk intensifies:

- "I used to be fast/strong/lean...now look at me."

- "What's the point when I'll never PR again?"

- "I'm just too tired all the time for early morning runs anymore."

Throw in disruptive symptoms like hot flashes or bladder leaks mid-workout and your confidence tanks further. You start questioning whether pursuing fitness still warrants priority status.

Here too, adjusting unrealistic expectations proves crucial given your changed reality. Setting pride aside to modify training, fuel properly, practice self-compassion and rally

your why connects the dots ensuring you continue moving -
even if workouts look different from the glory days.

Modifying Fitness Strategies

Now that we've outlined the key impacts of menopause on
athletic performance, where do we go from here? How do
you maintain consistency with healthy movement to uphold
bone density, heart health, strength and resilience through
your transition?

Here are 5 broad guidelines to adapt fitness routines:

1. **Listen to your body** - Scale all training elements like
   volume, intensity and recovery windows according to
   symptoms and energy levels.

2. **Prioritize recovery** - Incorporate more mild active
   recovery days plus nourish muscles well with protein,
   healthy fats and micronutrients.

3. **Commit to strength training** - Offset muscle loss
   and hormonal shifts exacerbating injuries through 2-3
   weekly strength sessions.

4. **Go harder on nutrition** - Eliminate empty calories
   and inflammatory foods undermining training
   response.

5. **Redefine success** – Celebrate capability over
   comparison; consistency over PRs.

Let's break down specifics on tailoring methodology,
workout programming, nutrition support and mindset shifts
for this season of change.

Methodology Adjustments

Regarding broad stroke workout structure, consider these common modifications:

- Sub out one higher intensity session a week for extra active recovery like yoga, walking or easy cycling

- Shorten session duration slightly if hit by fatigue or losing focus

- Limit high impact, plyometric or extremely grinding sessions

- Practice active isolation stretching post-workout to increase pliability

Listen closely each day to joints, nagging pains or low energy cues indicating when to pull back intensity, duration or training load to support recovery. Remain consistent showing up with 80% effort on days you feel blah still nets benefits long term over skipping workouts or not fueling properly.

Program Tweaks

In terms of training plan specifics, these modifications help avoid overuse injuries and stagnation:

- Build progression through volume increases before intensity bumps

- Cycle between 2 weeks hard training then 1 week active recovery

- Balance heavy pressing with plenty posterior chain work *Perform single leg exercises reducing shear forces

- Include Pilates, Gyrotonics or other offset loads

Emphasize strength and stability over cardio dependent improvement during the menopausal transition. Support whatever aerobic activity energizes you but don't stress paces or output declining in running, cycling or similar sports.

Nutrition Support

Doubling down on high quality nutrition prevents backsliding too much from unavoidable metabolic shifts. Here's how to fuel for fitness during menopause:

- Meet daily protein needs - up to 1 gram per pound of body weight - to prevent muscle wasting

- Load anti-inflammatory foods like fatty fish, colorful produce, nuts and olive oil

- Hydrate really well, especially in summer months

- Eliminate refined carbs and added sugars dragging down energy

- Consider supplements like omega-3s, vitamin D, calcium, collagen and magnesium

Eat plenty of wholesome nourishing foods so your hard training doesn't go to waste. Monitor macro ratios to keep protein adequate relative to carbohydrate intake.

Mindset Tips

Finally, stay motivated through inevitable ebbs and flows using these psychological tips:

- Cultivate self-compassion for off days

- Focus on consistency over continually progressing

- Define success by subjective enjoyment vs objective metrics

- Surround yourself with supportive community

- Remind yourself change remains temporary

You've got this! With knowledge plus personalized modifications, the menopausal fitness transition doesn't have to derail your goals. Expect ups and downs while celebrating little victories like recovery run breakthroughs or hitting milestones like pullup numbers. Your strong capable body still holds pleasant surprises even amidst hormonal chaos.

Knowing What to Expect

Wrapping up our foundation of menopausal physiology, let's tie everything together on what to expect as your body transitions through perimenopause, reaches menopause and continues adjusting afterwards.

While each woman's experience varies dramatically, overviews help you anticipate changes down the line. Consider this chapter your crystal ball glimpse of what's to come and when so you feel empowered, not blindsided.

We'll cover:

- Common Symptom Timeline

- Expected Changes by Life Stage

- Setting Appropriate Expectations *Seeking Support When Needed

Here's the birdseye view of the winding menopausal road ahead.

Typical Perimenopause & Menopause Symptom Timeline

Though individual timing and severity differs, most women traverse a similar order of events through perimenopause into established menopause:

Early Stage Perimenopause

- Periods grow irregular - longer, shorter or inconsistent cycles

- Light spotting between periods

- PMS symptoms intensify - bloating, cramps, heavy bleeding

- Fatigue, trouble sleeping and mood changes emerge

- Weight creeps up inexplicably

Mid-Late Stage Perimenopause

- Very long - 60+ days or very short - 21 days cycles

- First hot flashes or night sweats appear

- Vaginal dryness less responsive to lubricants

- Urinary urgency or leakage issues

- Increased insomnia, anxiety, forgetfulness, brain fog

Menopause Year

- Last menstrual period - cue red wine 🍷

- Most disruptive hot flashes peak

- Blood sugar regulation, cholesterol changes intensify

- Postmenopause bone loss accelerates after final period

- Vulnerability rises for heart disease and diabetes

- Symptoms feel unrelenting before stabilizing

Early Postmenopause

- Finally hot flashes decrease bout 1 year after last period

- Intensity of symptoms gradually improve

- Sex drive, arousal and satisfaction issues persist

- Sleep improves but often remains disrupted

- Joint pain, brain fog take longer to resolve

Long Term Postmenopause

- Most symptoms fade significantly by year 5 after final period

- Estrogen deficiency effects like bone loss continue long term

- Disease vulnerability persists without proper lifestyle steps

- Aging manifests faster without estrogen benefits

Obviously the menopause transition extends far longer with more nuance than most women first realize so update your expectations accordingly! The intensity of symptoms often plateaus a couple years then improves. Let's examine typical changes unfolding across different life stages too.

What to Expect by Life Stage

Beyond the progressive sequence of menstrual cycle changes then settlement into postmenopause, your experience also varies based on phases of parenthood along with career and caregiving variables.

Women struggling through demanding stretches with young kids at home or aging parents to assist often battle intensified anxiety, overwhelm and exhaustion compared to empty nesters with more bandwidth for self care. Stress management rivals addressing physiological symptoms.

Likewise physical activity and nutrition habits surge or suffer based on work deadlines or leisure time freedom as kids transition toward independence. Compare a mom driving kids to evening activities ping-ponging between school meetings and domestic duties with a woman enjoying regular morning bike rides and abundant quiet evenings for meal prep.

The following snapshots capture "typical" symptom manifestations and self-care realities through milestone decades:

Perimenopause - 40s

- Often exhausting stage of parenting, domestic and career responsibilities. Difficulty determining cause of fatigue or weight gain between lifestyle and hormone changes. Too busy to slow down so push through symptoms.

- Once recognize perimenopause shift, hard to prioritize self care between many obligations. Counseling or support groups help overwhelmed caregiver stress. Can't eliminate stressful trigger so focus relief tactics through transition years.

- Symptom severity seems unfair added onto demanding life stretch but does improve overtime. Celebrate milestones like kids gaining independence or work projects ending also lightening load.

Menopause - Late 40s-Early 50s

- Worst symptoms like intense hot flashes, unraveling sleep and low libido hopefully hit during a less hectic life season offering more bandwidth for self care. If kids don't need shuttling to constant activities or parents require less hands on support, take advantage focusing more inward now.

- Make time for things like yoga, supplements, nutritious cooking or couples connection if possible amidst the discomfort or emotional volatility flaring up currently from hormone chaos.

- Set intentions embracing this transition as springboard for second act dreams not a backwards slide. Maybe you downshift career wise or return to postponed creative, athletic or travel pursuits without feeling guilty. Fertility winding down frees you up for long deferred goals. What whispers now from your empowered inner wisdom?

Postmenopause - 50s and Beyond

- With demanding reproductive years transitioning behind you and freedom from periods, birth control side effects, early parenthood challenges etc, direct energy towards revitalized goals for this next stage. What hobbies, adventures or bucket list dreams capture your spirit?

- By a few years after the intensity of hot flashes, vaginal dryness and similar symptoms improve, you can fully focus forward without menopause drama stealing mental bandwidth. Regained energy and emotional equilibrium arrives right as you have more space for long deferred or newfound passions. Channel positivity!

- Commit to lifestyle habits cementing health and vitality for vibrant decades ahead now. Whether continuing established fitness routines or trying new modalities like dance, make self care priority before aging accelerates. Inspire other women through vulnerability, wisdom and confidence on the other side!

Hopefully these snapshots help calibrate expectations about what you'll likely struggle with or look forward to during different phases of winding down fertility into freedom. Sympathy and solutions await no matter what level of chaos or calm your personal menopause experience brings in coming years. You've got this!

Setting Appropriate Expectations

Beyond anticipating what a "typical" menopausal timeline entails by life stage, we all must keep expectations flexible given huge individual variability. Comparing your situation too strictly against norms or friends often backfires. Give yourself permission for a unique experience!

For instance if you previously sailed through pregnancy, childbirth and periods effortlessly yet now suffer severe hot flashes, mood swings and pain during perimenopause, don't panic. Just because discomfort feels foreign doesn't mean something is terribly wrong or that agony will persist permanently. How our bodies respond now doesn't necessarily follow previous paths.

Likewise if you've struggled for years managing endometriosis, fibroid pain or heavy periods making you dread cycles, don't automatically assume menopause will intensify previous issues. You may breeze by relatively unscathed!

Remain cautiously optimistic in all cases. Don't fret endlessly or catastrophize worst case scenarios if symptoms hit hard for now. This too shall pass! Likewise don't toss out discipline around healthy habits prematurely believing you've already endured the worst. Skimping on fitness, nutrition, stress management or self care during early postmenopause often backfires when vulnerability persists.

Adopting balanced expectations allows appropriately preparing and preventing struggles yet also receiving each stage openly without preconceived limitations on what's possible for your experience.

Seeking Support When Needed

Finally, remember that while all women endure the menopause marathon to some degree, nobody needs run solo! Reach out for professional support or community wisdom when the path feels too rocky.

No shame exists in needing extra assistance whether physically, emotionally or psychologically during transitions. We all face challenges better together.

Consider seeking help from the following sources if you experience:

- Depression, overwhelming anxiety or emotional volatility disrupting work, relationships or daily life

- Hot flashes, insomnia or similar symptoms continually preventing restful sleep and functioning

- Painful sex, vaginal atrophy or urinary incontinence deteriorating intimacy or quality of life

- Rapid, concerning weight gain or nutritional deficits

- Debilitating joint pain preventing basic activity

- Feelings of grief, resentment or hopelessness during the menopausal transition

Support looks different for everyone from asking your gynecologist about menopausal health, booking appointments with a registered dietitian, signing up for talk therapy or joining a support group.

Know that while fluctuating hormone changes eventually stabilize after menopause, caring well for whole self shouldn't wait indefinitely if you feel overwhelmed in the present. You deserve help now, not just comfort later when symptoms pass. Reach out!

In Summary

Hopefully this advice prepares you to anticipate menopause related changes rolling through life's different stages. I aim for you to feel informed, empowered and supported for the transition ahead based on education around what typically unfolds plus permission to write your own story.

Remember your menopausal process follows no "right" script. Let go of comparing yourself to friends or family, release fears magnifying worst case scenarios and proceed through phases utilizing resources as needed. You've got this!

Part II: Optimizing Your Wellbeing

Now that you understand the physiology behind what's happening during the menopausal transition, let's move onto practical solutions easing symptoms for greater comfort, happiness and wellbeing as your hormone levels shift.

Consider Part II your tactical guide covering science-backed lifestyle "hacks" along with medical and holistic interventions to customize relief. We'll address managing common disruptive issues like:

- Hot flashes, night sweats and improving sleep

- Physical discomforts - vaginal dryness, bladder problems, joint pain, headaches

- Low energy, brain fog, mood swings and emotional challenges

- Weight gain, cardiovascular disease, osteoporosis and other health risks

Beyond treating symptomatic struggles, we'll dig deeper into optimizing nutrition, fitness, mindset and self care practices for renewing vitality. Think thriving not just surviving!

Too often women simply suffer through menopausal misery believing little can be done or that wine and icy stares from irritated partners represent their only coping tools. Not so ladies!

From tapping into the wisdom traditions like ayurveda and Traditional Chinese Medicine to learning practical clean eating upgrades from registered dietitians, you're about to discover pages of little known hacks and innovative interventions helping you feel balanced in body and mind again.

Consider this section your awakening...Yes to feeling great in your skin joyfully living your purpose no matter what date appears on the calendar! No to stagnating unconsciously at the mercy of temporary hormone changes. The vibrant you awaits rediscovered. Flip the page to begin!

Managing Hot Flashes, Night Sweats & More

Kicking off tactics for optimizing wellness through the menopausal transition, let's start with the symptoms disrupting comfort and quality of life most notoriously - hot flashes and night sweats. Up to 80% of women experience them from early perimenopause into postmenopause until hormone levels stabilize, so you're not alone!

This chapter explains exactly what causes hot flashes along with night sweats and related issues like chills, flushing, headache, anxiety and more. You'll discover science-backed solutions medicinal and lifestyle based for preventing and minimizing severity of heat waves when they strike.

We'll cover natural remedies, nutrition and fitness interventions, prescription options, mindfulness practices and environmental tweaks bringing relief on multiple fronts. Arm yourself with diverse tools to cool down those temporary infernos and manage related discomforts so you can carry on living fully while flashes run their course.

What Causes Hot Flashes & Night Sweats?

As introduced earlier, hot flashes result from declining estrogen levels interacting with your hypothalamus - the body's temperature regulation center in the brain. Declining estrogen sensitizes the hypothalamus, causing it to overreact releasing signals triggering blood vessels near skin to rapidly dilate then quickly constrict again.

This surge of blood flow heats skin prompting sweating to cool the body back down once the hypothalamic hot flash episode concludes. Night sweats follow the same mechanism, just occurring while sleeping which often wakes women up.

Triggers range from warm environments, stress, spicy foods, alcohol or caffeine to surprise factors you can't pinpoint. Often came on out of nowhere it seems! Generally alleviating lifestyle triggers and supporting healthy circulation with nutrition supplements and mindfulness practices helps prevent onset. Managing environment, layers and hydration offsets severity once hot flashes strike.

Lifestyle, Natural Remedies & Nutrition Support

Let's begin relieving hot flash misery through lifestyle upgrades and evidence based natural remedies before considering medical intervention:

1. Identify & Avoid Triggers

Keep a diary tracking when hot flashes happen, severity, how long they last plus suspected trigger factors like stress, food or drink you had recently. Look for patterns about timing, triggers and relieving factors based on your entries. Avoid common triggers when possible.

2. Layer Light Breathable Fabrics

Dress in thin moisture wicking layers you can remove as needed rather than thick fabrics trapping heat yet provide quick cover for chill phase after a hot flash. keeping shoulders or neck area cool may help prevent some flushes too.

3. Lower Ambient Temperature

Keep your overall household thermostat a bit cooler and use small fans as needed to improve air circulation and cooling during a hot flash. Cooling wrist bands, freeze therapy vests and other products help too.

4. Hydrate Well With Electrolytes

Stay hydrated with mineral rich fluids like coconut water and herbal iced tea versus just plain water to replace salts and nutrients lost from sweating. Infused waters with fruit, cucumbers or herbs tantalize your tastebuds too.

5. Avoid Caffeine, Alcohol & Spicy Foods

All three of those popular indulgences can trigger hot flashes so use sparingly if at all while you navigate menopause symptoms.

6. Consider Soy, Black Cohosh or Vitamin E

Clinical trials found minimal/mixed evidence that supplements like soy isoflavones, black cohosh and vitamin E alleviate hot flashes but some women do experience relief from them. Dosage around 50-100 mgs isoflavones or black cohosh daily appears most promising if you want to experiment under healthcare supervision.

7. Practice Deep Breathing

When you feel a hot flash creeping up, get into rest pose either standing or sitting comfortably. Close your eyes and take long slow deep inhales through your nose followed by extended exhales through barely parted lips for at least 60 seconds. This relaxation response lowers stress hormones that can trigger flushing onset.

8. Boost Circulation With Nitrates

Foods rich in nitrates like arugula, beets and pomegranate may improve vascular responsiveness helping prevent hot flash intensity. More research needed but easy to add servings to your diet.

9. Balance Blood Sugar

Eating frequent small meals with nutrient dense whole food carbohydrates while avoiding added sugars and refined flour stabilizes blood glucose highs and lows. This prevents energy crashes, mood swings or headaches that exacerbate hot flashes.

10. Consider Acupuncture

Some research indicates acupuncture successfully reduces hot flash frequency and severity for menopausal women. Work with a licensed practitioner targeting meridians involved with circulation and body temperature regulation for best results.

Lifestyle remedies should help decrease the intensity of hot flashes and night sweats even if not eliminating them completely in early phases. If you experience minimal relief or very disruptive symptoms after a few months implementing changes, consider adding medical support.

When To Ask Your Doctor About Prescriptions

If hot flashes or night sweats disrupt sleep, work performance or quality of life after diligently applying natural remedies, consult your healthcare provider about adding medications for relief. Especially reach out promptly if you struggle with mood changes like depression or extreme irritability and anxiety exacerbating your situation.

Prescription and over the counter options range from hormonal treatments replacing estrogen, antidepressants and anticonvulsants calming nervous system reactions to herbal blends with clinical research supporting benefits.

Doctors often prescribe the lowest dose over shortest duration possible balancing benefits against potential health risks of added hormones or medications during the menopausal transition. Work closely monitoring your response.

Hormone therapy (HT) replaces estrogen with a patch, pill, cream, ring, shot or pellet implant aiming to stabilize hormones related to temperature regulation thus cooling hot flashes. Localized ultra low dose vaginal estrogen creams treat genitourinary issues rather than whole body systems.

How long until HT alleviates your hot flashes? Consistent use decreases frequency around 70% within 1 month for most women and continues improving effects to about a 90% reduction at 6 months. Many wean off HT after worst symptoms pass as hormones rebalance naturally by 1-5 years after menopause

SSRIs like low dose fluoxetine or citalopram modulate serotonin and other brain chemicals providing non hormonal hot flash relief likely by modulating temperature regulating pathways. Similarly **SNRIs**, antiseizure meds and herbal blends influence nerve pathways.

Gabapentin treats neuralgia nerve pain from shingles, diabetes or injury. Off label applications at low 300mg/day dosage calms hot flash symptoms for 60-70% of women not responding fully to lifestyle remedies or preferring non hormones.

Clonidine lowers blood pressure by smoothing vascular responses. The 0.1 mg pill also reduces hot flash frequency and severity around 40-50% as a side effect by blocking adrenaline surges. Constipation and drowsiness occur as frequent unwanted side effects however.

Hopefully exploring a diversity of evidenced based conventional plus complementary options bolsters your toolbox relieving temporary misery from common menopause symptoms until your body chemistry stabilizes in the months following your final period. Now let's cover other discomforts beyond hot flashes impacting quality of life.

Conclusion - What To Do About Other Physical Symptoms

Like hot flashes, night sweats and similar troubling issues, most other physical discomforts women endure through perimenopause and early post menopause fortunately tend to run their course over time as hormones recalibrate at lower levels. Trust their impermanence even on rough days!

However lasting relief awaits by proactively targeting lifestyle remedies and therapeutic interventions providing symptom management until the phase passes.

We'll cover specific solutions for concerns like:

- Painful intercourse, vaginal dryness and urinary tract infections

- Weight gain, blood sugar dysregulation and nutrition tactics

- Brain fog, memory lapses, mood swings and emotional volatility

- Insomnia and sleep disturbances

- Joint pain, stiffness and mobility issues

Take comfort, you can alleviate frustrating symptoms through nutrition upgrades, fitness modifications, stress relief practices and strategic supplementation even if some stubborn discomforts linger longer than you desire. This too shall pass!

Supporting Bone, Brain, Heart & Immune Health

With a solid understanding now about what drives common disruptive menopause symptoms and solutions providing relief, let's pivot to safeguarding overall wellness for thriving long term even after fertility winds down.

I want to equip you to proactively care for key body systems like bone, brain, heart and immune health using nutrition, fitness and lifestyle upgrades minimizing heightened risks for chronic diseases as estrogen production sputters out. Consider this your owners manual for operating an aging vehicle strategically!

We'll cover:

- Bone loss threats and prevention tactics

- Keeping your brain sharp, energized and stable

- Guarding cardiovascular and metabolic health

- Supporting immunity and cellular renewal

- Integrative approaches leveraging Eastern traditions

Just like a car requires extra maintenance checking fluids, tightening belts and replacing worn parts over decades to keep rolling smoothly down the road of life, our bodies need added care over time too!

Let's get to those crucial pitstops ensuring you live vibrantly for years to come.

Stopping Bone Loss in Its Tracks

Starting with skeletal health, estrogens key role building bone density until around age 30 then helping maintain bone strength by regulating the constant turnover between bone building osteoblasts and bone resorbing osteoclasts means dropping estrogen levels after menopause accelerate bone mineral loss.

Left unchecked, gradual depletion coined osteopenia leads to full blown osteoporosis and greater fracture risks which no woman wants!

Begin getting ahead in early perimenopause before rapid loss starts by:

1.**Getting a baseline bone density DEXA scan** – This special Xray allows tracking the health of your bones over time detecting osteopenia or osteoporosis early when you have decades more to halt damage and even rebuild lost density through proper interventions. Most women should start scans around age 50.

2.**Consume at least 1200mg calcium daily** - From dairy products, leafy greens, nuts and supplements as needed to provide essential building blocks keeping bones mineralized and strong.

3.**Take 1000-4000 IU Vitamin D3** - The "sunshine" nutrient plays a pivotal role regulating calcium absorption and bone building cell activity. Optimal levels around 40-60 ng/mL associate with greater bone density.

4.**Incorporate weight bearing and resistance training** 2-3 times per week – Exercises bearing body weight and adding heavy loads through free weights, machines, Pilates devices or other tools stimulate bone strengthening just like muscle development. Walking doesn't provide enough load.

5.**Monitor status and medicate if needed** – Repeat DEXA scans every 1-3 years allow your doctor to determine if bone densities drop into concerning ranges warranting prescription bisphosphonates like Fosamax or Prolia, hormone therapy etc under medical supervision.

6.**Consider newer bone building alternatives** - Cutting edge therapies show promise too like peptide Ostera stimulating osteoblasts, parathyroid hormone Forteo or bone antiresorptive Romosozumab if first line meds don't maintain densities.

Committing earlier to bone building and protecting strategies leverages the window before estrogen levels bottom out to mitigate destruction and safeguards your strong capable frame carrying you through elder years fracture free!

Let's pivot to equally important neurological health and cognitive function defense.

Keeping Your Brain Sharp

Simultaneously structural brain changes along with complex intersections between estrogen, stress hormones, inflammation, genetics and cardiovascular issues set the stage for cognitive declines, memory lapses and mood instability risks to increase after menopause.

Outsmart these threats by:

1.**Exercising your mind** – Just like physical muscles, keep your neurological pathways strong through continual learning. Read books, take classes, do crossword puzzles, diversify hobbies to keep your brain's plasticity high.

2.**Committing to regular workouts** – What's good for your heart proves great for your head too. Starting simple walking routines pays exponential dividends keeping brain blood flow and structural connections optimized.

3.**Loading up on anti-inflammatory "brain foods"** like fatty fish, colorful berries and dark chocolate driving down oxidative stress damage, improve signaling, support gut microbes tied to mental health and maintain fluid membrane integrity protecting neurons.

4.**Optimizing key supplements** like omega 3s from fish oils boosting BDNF brain growth factors, magnesium easing anxiety and nervous system hyperactivity, B vitamins fueling nerve transmission and more based on lab testing if levels show low/borderline.

5.**Managing stress effectively** – From sufficient sleep, nature immersion, yoga, laughter, counseling or whatever activities elicit your relaxation response counteracts damage from cortisol, adrenaline and inflammation that cripples brain structure and chemistry when elevated chronically.

Fortify your thinking organ daily because just like heart health, Tomorrow's vibrant cognition depends on Today's consistent loving action to nourish this vital body system. Let's cover cardiac & metabolic health next.

Guarding Cardiovascular & Metabolic Health

As introduced earlier, lowered estrogen correlates to adverse cholesterol changes, elevated inflammation and vascular responsiveness plus higher blood sugars that together drive up heart disease and diabetes risks for postmenopausal women.

You are in no way destined for disease however! Again lifestyle choices wield mighty influence preventing illness in elder decades despite unavoidable hormone related vulnerabilities.

Your action plan for robust circulation and metabolism includes:

1.**Achieve or maintain optimal body composition** – Carrying excess body fat directly contributes to inflammatory cytokine production, insulin resistance, cholesterol ratio imbalances and cardiovascular strain. Strategically support healthy calorie burning muscle and steady nourishing metabolism through training, nutrition and sleep.

2.**Incorporate 30-60 minutes daily moderate+ activity** – Whatever you enjoy that keeps your heart rate elevated - walking, riding, dancing etc. Shoot for at least 150 minutes weekly minimum for disease protection.

3.**Eat anti-inflammatory whole foods** – Abundantly nourish yourself with produce colors, fiber diversity, healthy fats from nuts/avocados/olive oil, fatty fish and probiotic support from fermented foods/supplements while limiting added sugars, refined grains and pro-inflammatory industrialized oils.

4.**Monitor blood biomarkers annually** - Keep tabs on fasting glucose, HbA1c percentages, triglycerides, LDL, HDL and total cholesterol. Metformin, statins or prescription estrogen may assist if levels indicate high risk after lifestyle changes.

Like with building bone density, earlier committed action securing ideal heart and metabolic markers pays exponential dividends later as hormone related threats increase with age. But remember even 75 year old women demonstrate cardiovascular adaptation and diabetes risk reduction through initiating exercise, food upgrades and body composition improvement - it just takes longer compared to being proactive at menopause onset. Don't wait!

Finally let's touch on supporting immunity, energy production and cellular health.

Bolstering Immunity, Energy & Cellular Health

Aging inevitably involves gradual physiological decline across body systems. Yet the speed at which our cells, mitochondria and internal defense systems decay depends largely on environmental exposures and lifestyle choices.

You can absolutely slow deterioration, nourish vitality and even demonstrate biomarkers of more youthful health deep into your elder decades by:

1.**Relentlessly striving for 8+ hours nightly sleep** in cool, pitch black settings allowing deep restorative states rejuvenating immunity and cellular repair.

2.**Reducing exposure to toxins** that disrupt delicate hormonal pathways, overwhelm liver detoxification systems and damage DNA like industrial chemicals in skin care or household products, air pollution, molds etc. Eliminate threats within your control.

3.**Hydrating optimally** with clean pure water and mineral rich fluids delivering nutrients into cells and flushing waste products out.

4.**Eating abundant antioxidant foods** like deeply colored produce boasting polyphenols and anthocyanins neutralizing free radical damage accumulating from stresses while also supporting natural glutathione production and metalloproteinases guarding telomeres.

5.**Investigating functional supplements** like NAD+ boosters, spermidine and resveratrol that rodent studies show extend lifespan by as much as 15% by activating gene expression pathways regulating aging though human evidence remains scant currently. Can't hurt adding a few!

Remember, while some bodily performance decline proves inevitable (you can't entirely halt aging!), how rapidly head to toe deterioration unfolds directly relates to nutrition status, fitness consistency, mindset priority and environmental exposures.

You absolutely wield power influencing the difference between disability at 65 versus still hand standing on a yoga mat at 85! Body, brain and spirit - take care of this temple daily.

Eastern Traditions For Renewal

Beyond conventional western tactics supporting menopausal health and wellbeing, integrative modalities from traditional Chinese medicine and India's ancient Ayurvedic system also provide wisdom guiding this transition.

Ayurveda recognizes the doshas - combinations of elemental forces represented by vata, pitta and kapha. Declining estrogen exaggerates already prevalent vata characteristics in most middle aged women like dryness, anxiety, lightness, irregularity and forgetfulness.

Counsel your inner balance through opposites - choosing grounding, nourishing, slow, warm and heavy activities. Favor sweet, sour and salty foods over bitter, astringent and pungent while emphasizing stable rhythms. All counteract heightened vata dosha.

Traditional Chinese Medicine views menopause as depletion of yin fluids and blood exacerbating already ascendant yang energies that comes with age. Symptoms like hot flashes and vaginal dryness stem from kidney yin deficiency failing to balance heart yang surges. Acupuncture, herbs and lifestyle changes nourish Yin.

Both systems emphasize restoration through food, mindful movement and self care - we just discussed in conventional terms the importance circulation support, stress reduction, bone building, antioxidant nourishment etc. Integrating traditional wisdom expands tactical options personalized to your constitution.

Hopefully reviewing key vulnerabilities of brain, bone, cardiovascular and immune health during the menopausal transition along with lifestyle remedies from both eastern and western vantage points empowers you to take positive steps forward. Prioritize daily action setting you up for success!

Sleep, Stress & Self Care Strategies

Moving beyond specifically menopause related health risks into broader wellness pillars, let's address crucial lifestyle factors affecting overall quality of life greatly during midlife transition years - sleep, stress management and self care.

Poor sleep proves nearly universal disturbing up to 60% of perimenopausal and menopausal women with hot flashes and night sweats usually copping most blame. However, equally pressing roots of insomnia, fragmented rest and suboptimal sleep hygiene relate to habits around work life balance, technology usage, alcohol or caffeine indulgences plus psychological overload - especially salient issues midlife women face.

Without adequate sleep cascading impacts cripple nearly every body system compromising mental health, metabolic health, immunity, injury resistance, emotional regulation, relationship harmony and more. Prioritizing restorative sleep and balanced stress responses pays exponential dividends during chaotic hormonal years and beyond. This chapter explains why along with tactical tips improving sleep, moods and resilience even amidst menopausal chaos.

Sleep & Menopause

We all intuitively grasp sleep equals key for health. Yet shockingly 75% of Americans report consistent rest troubles while only 3% meet clinical sleep health standards of uninterrupted quality slumber adding up to the 7-9 hour minimum most adults require. Quantity and quality both matter hugely.

Among menopausal women already facing turmoil from hot flashes, stress and potential mood disorders, depleted sleep exacerbates every symptom while also undermining disease prevention efforts around fitness, nutrition and self care adherence. Vicious cycles ensue tanking work productivity, relationship harmony, weight management plus optimism when nights pass fitfully.

Beyond temporary solutions like sleeping pills, stress reducers or cognitive behavioral therapy easing insomnia, we must better understand sleep phases along with evidenced based facets of sleep hygiene positively influencing nightly rest quality. Master these fundamentals setting the stage for lifelong wellbeing through and beyond the menopausal marathon.

Phases of Sleep

Sleep unfolds in predictable patterns cycling through light, deep and REM stages a handful of times per night. Each phase serves restoration needs. Trouble arises when we don't traverse every stage enough times or stay disrupted by awakenings.

Non-REM Light Sleep occupies initial descent first transitioning from alert beta brain waves into beginning alpha and theta dreaming activity accompanied by slightly lowered heart rate and body temperature. Healthy sleep requires 10-25% here but no more than 50%.

Non-REM Deep Sleep follows marked by the slow delta brain waves pulsing maximum tissue recovery, immunity strengthening, memory solidifying and metabolic harmony flowing. This rebuilds your body best hitting 20-40% of total overnight sleep.

REM (Rapid Eye Movement) benefits culminate each 90-minute cycle featuring vivid dreams, muscle paralysis and spiky brain activity while repair hormones like HGH and testosterone peak. Emotional healing happens reaching 20-25% total REM with 4-6 stage cycles overnight.

Ideally, we traverse all phases multiple times without waking for sufficient mind, body and soul nourishing rest although many factors like lifestyle choices and underlying health conditions disrupt hygiene. As we age particularly, deep and REM sleep stages often suffer.

While temporary medication like sleeping pills appear seductive for desperate insomnia, chronic use proves counterproductive since chemical alterations prevent reaching reparative slow wave and REM states critical for cognitive sharpness and emotional health. You miss out on essential restoration!

Sleep Hygiene Fundamentals

Improving sleep thrives not through pills but optimizing daily habits dictating nightly capacity to fully dive through every cycle. Below we'll cover key lifestyle sleep hygiene categories to overhaul starting today.

Reduce Evening Blue Light - manmade lighting tricks biology. Screens on phones/tablets/TVs emit high intensity blue wavelengths communicating "daytime!" to master circadian pathways so they don't release our natural sedating melatonin at appropriate evening hours. Limit exposure especially before bed.

Keep Consistent Bed/Wake Hours - chaotic schedules confuse circadian signals also dampening melatonin release and keep sleep/wake brain centers from fully switching modes overnight. Even weekends try stick 8 hours total in same time window.

Make Your Bedroom A Sanctuary - cool, dark and gadget free zones avoid overstimulation. Blackout curtains, ear plugs if noisy, blue light blocking glasses and no scrolling while in this sacred space. Let cues signal rest awaiting here.

Establish Soothing Wind Down Rituals - journaling, stretching, meditation or skincare regimens in the 90 minutes before lights out begin triggering relaxation responses preparing mind and body for slumber instead of ruminating about stressors.

Avoid Unsupportive Substances - limit caffeine after noon, cap alcohol before bed and ditch inflammatory refined carbs/sugars spiking then crashing energy. Support natural cycles instead with herbal tea, magnesium rich foods and yoga. You'll sleep and wake better.

Consider Chronotherapy - gradually shifting bedtime earlier by 15 minutes every few nights recalibrates overactive alarm clock centers thrown off when insomnia persists long term. Eases falling asleep again without medication dependence.

See Your Doctor - rule out contributing factors like sleep apnea, restless legs or hormone imbalances. Maybe adjustment to existing medications or brief therapy for racing thoughts allows sleeping soundly again. Don't accept tough nights as inevitable before exploring solutions.

Prioritizing restorative sleep provides the ultimate foundation handling stressful life seasons gracefully while also supporting every OTHER health and wellbeing goal optimally. Keep this your number one non negotiable self care pillar above even fitness or nutrition efforts which inevitably suffer if operating chronically sleep deprived. Nighty night!

Stress Management & Emotional Health

No woman navigates perimenopause or the years surrounding your final period unscathed by stress, uncertainty and cascading lifestyle changes affecting family, career, identity, health or relationships. Add mood fluctuations from hormone changes plus sleep volatility and no wonder anxiety and emotional volatility soar for many!

Effective stress management serves as THE difference maker between barely surviving chaos until menopause passes or continuing to thrive while lean into changes courageously. Life presents sufficient challenges without piling on unnecessary suffering through unmanaged worries, mindset pitfalls or isolation.

We all endure pains, setbacks and fear on the lifelong path of growth. How you meet and process stressful experiences, treat yourself compassionately through missteps and leverage community connection amid adversity determines long-term empowerment.

Fortunately evidence based practices abound helping women gracefully dance through external life challenges and internal emotional triggers activated strongly at menopause:

Cultivate Perspective - view stressors (big or small annoyances) through a lens of growth opportunity. How might this experience shape my character positively? Seek meaning amidst the messy. Everything changes eventually - good and bad times too. Breathe easier knowing struggles pass.

Lean On Community - nobody succeeds solo! Give and receive support discussing issues with trusted friends who uplift and empower. Share feelings openly to release bottled up frustration or grief. Support groups filled with others navigating menopause build solidarity too.

Infuse Daily Fun - laugh, play, create, move or relax choosing enjoyable activities lowering stress hormone levels fast while boosting confidence to tackle problems. Even when crazy busy enjoy little pleasures like listening to comedy or music that makes you smile. Delight fuels resilience handling adversity.

Practice Mindfulness - train redirecting attention constantly to the present moment rather than obsessing past regrets or future worries through mantras, meditation, yoga or any hobby absorbing focus totally. Detach thoughts from inevitable judgements building more spacious mindset relief.

Improve Self Talk - notice tendency towards pessimistic explanations focusing blame inward and shift dialogue gently towards more accurate understanding of situations with compassion for yourself and others. We all struggle sometimes so cut slack!

Arm yourself with diverse stress management practices above along with sufficient nourishing sleep optimizing capacity staying emotionally and mentally even keeled through the menopause marathon plus any other life storms ahead. Your balanced outlook underpins health. Now we'll tie together key tenets of self care guaranteed enhancing wellbeing as estrogen wanes.

Self Care Fundamentals

We've covered extensively proper nutrition, consistent training, restorative sleep and stress relief as cornerstones guarding overall menopausal health. Now let's connect how mastering self-care fundamentals makes implementing those pillars sustainable when Bonaparte life circumstances still strain even our best laid plans.

Lackluster fitness consistency, poor dietary adherence or skimping on sleep rarely happen due to simple laziness but instead stem from depleted mental bandwidth handling too many priorities simultaneously. Self-care forms centerpiece to your entire wellbeing foundation. Get this right and everything else flows more effortlessly!

But what is self-care actually beyond just pampering moments like massages or bubble baths? The essence equates to prioritizing emotional, physical and spiritual health DAILY through any actions nurturing your best self so you confidently and energetically show up, achieving goals. SKIP

Strategic self- care involves:

Defining Your Core Values - determining personal standards and boundaries guiding all decisions removes excuse making and distractions pulling you off purpose for health. Live aligned and there will be no inner conflict sapping mental strength better spent pursuing passions.

Mastering Stress Mindset - reframe how you view obstacles emotionally as explained above. Adopting growth opportunity perspective minimizes wasted energy resisting the universal fact that problems will always arise. Stress becomes far less ominous.

Establishing Reward Systems - attach pleasurable incentives along the sometimes challenging path of building new habits or refusing unhealthy temptations that compromise willpower. Link small treats to your values like a massage after 30 days perfect gym attendance or fancy coffee date with friends if you pass on wine temptations for a week. Move towards inspiration.

Make no mistake, self-care abilities prove especially imperative when facing social, emotional or physical stressors depleting mental reserves and sabotaging motivation like those perimenopause and menopause oft accompany. Rectifying inadequate self-care habits change every game. Tune inward to your deepest soul truths and live aligned with courage positive conviction!

Healthy Weight Maintenance

By now you're well aware from hormone happenings to lifestyle shifts how menopause transitions present unique challenges losing weight or halting subtle middle age creep of padding despite consistent healthy habits. Declining metabolism, rising hunger signals, sweet cravings and systemic inflammation all collude piling pounds where we want them least!

But just as clearly the importance minimizing excess body fat supports nearly every aspect of wellness — appearance confidence, training performance, sexual health, disease prevention and beyond — during midlife and entering elder decades. Excess adiposity cripples health by fueling inflammation and destroying metabolic harmony contributing greatly to diabetes, dementia, fatty liver, stroke, heart attack and cancer risks. Meanwhile fitness and vitality decline.

The urgency around maintaining ideal weight through menopause cannot be overstated even as biology fights against us! So beyond just commiserating struggles, let's get you answers why the scale climbs plus proven strategies reversing momentum for body composition victory entering your vibrant second act. This chapter explains what specifically happens hormonally and metabolically during peri and postmenopause facilitating fat storage along with key interventions counteracting weight gain.

Why Weight Loss Grows Harder

Everyone notices metabolism slowing down year after year even with consistent nutrition and training habits in place. Annual weight creep results as we age and that slog turns into utter sabotage after menopause if not strategically addressed through an estrogen aware gameplan. Here's why pounds add on more easily after midlife:

Loss of Estrogen directly stimulates fat storing enzymes in your abdominal area to activate while concurrently opposing mechanisms releasing stored fat break down. Your ovaries retiring promotes your belly holding onto every calorie for dear life! Making matters worse visceral belly fat secretes its own hormones impairing weight regulation further.

Increased Hunger & Cravings result from wonky hormonal crosstalk as reproductive hormones like progesterone also decline and stress hormones like cortisol increase. The hypothalamus gets bombarded by signals to seek quick energy from sweets and refined carbs especially at night disrupting the metabolic master switch.

Decreased Calorie Burn happens automatically because metabolically active muscle tissue burns far more energy pound for pound than fat. But our muscle mass percentage heads downhill after age 30 gradually, then falls off a cliff for a decade at menopause unless aggressively counteracted by strength training and adequate protein intake. Your resting metabolic engine downshifts accordingly.

Impaired Blood Sugar Regulation joins the party too as estrogen supports appropriate insulin release, triglycerides clearance and glycogen storage in youth which all falter during menopause. Glucose spikes faster but then lingers in your bloodstream longer thanks to insulin resistance promoting more belly fat accumulation and inflammatory damage.

In summary, menopause transitions present a dicey situation: you need fewer daily calories thanks to a slower metabolism and dwindling muscle mass yet feel hungrier more often while blood sugar and fat storing enzymes also go haywire. Losing or even just maintaining prior weight trends nearly impossible following old dietary approaches unless you understand WHAT to specifically modify and HOW to exercise optimizing hormones and metabolism uniquely for this season.

Fortunately you hold power to counteract the challenges! Now let's uncover solutions.

Winning Weight Loss Strategies

The same standard advice to "eat less and move more" falls devastatingly short (and discourages most women into despair) because that paradigm ignores our changed endocrine reality after menopause. You require strategic dietary composition supporting better blood sugar regulation and anabolic muscle building pathways in synergy with smart cardio and resistance training placing appropriate demand on tissues. Mindset adjustment helps too accepting gradual progress scaling small sustainable changes up over time replaces chasing extreme short term diets eventually backfiring.

We will overcome! Here are five pillars transforming your body composition and health trajectory for years ahead:

1) Moderate Carbohydrates

Eliminating added sugar remains mandatory (step one for everyone!) but next manage overall carbohydrate load keeping portions moderate and choosing complex whole food sources that benefit microbiome diversity like whole grains, starchy veggies and low glycemic fruits. Save sweets just for truly special occasions so insulin stays sensitized. About 40% carbs shoots optimal for menopausal women.

2) Prioritize Protein

To maintain precious calorie burning muscle mass as estrogen declines, protein intake deserves front seat hitting 20-30% total calories. Calculate needs at 1 gram per pound of target body weight daily from mixed complete sources like dairy, meat, fish, eggs, beans/legumes and supplemental collagen peptides or shakes. Spread protein across meals and before bed for sustained building, repair and hormonal support.

3) Healthy Fats Please

Beyond adequate protein also emphasize anti-inflammatory fats reaching 30-40% overall calories from olive oil, avocado, nuts/seeds, fatty fish and coconut products to provide steady energy, micronutrient absorption and joint protection. Ditch pro-inflammatory industrial seed oils! Enjoy olives, pesto, nut butters, salmon and full fat Greek yogurt.

4) Strength Train Most Days

Resistance training remains absolutely imperative to defend hard earned muscle mass as metabolism declines. Prioritize both upper and lower body work 2-3x weekly using moderately heavy loads for low reps to drive adaptation in nerves and muscle fibers. Squats, lunges step-ups and deadlifts (even bodyweight versions) work magic preventing thigh and glutes wasting! Don't just cardio.

5) Stress Less & Sleep More

You knew this one already too but cannot overemphasize how critical managing stress and securing 7-9 hours nightly sleep proves for optimizing weight regulation and health. Both habits minimize belly fat storage while decreasing inflammation, normalizing appetite signals and balancing key hormones that otherwise readily swing out of whack causing water retention, sugar crashes and rebound overeating.

While certain unwanted aesthetic and strength changes inevitably come for us all with age, you absolutely hold capacity stemming that downward trajectory through menopause and beyond by combining smarter nutrition that stabilizes hormones and fuels muscle recovery in synergy with consistent training spurring gains. Meet your body where it's at while also asking what it needs daily to continue gradually progressing. Small tweaks add up to big transformation in time. You've got this lady!

Building Your Support Squad

Wrapping up our wellbeing pillars for thriving through menopausal transitions, I want to acknowledge just how emotionally and physically taxing this journey proves for so many women. You may intellectually understand the physiology behind what's happening and tangibly implement lifestyle remedies yet still struggle feeling frustrated, isolated or doubtful amidst change.

You are not alone! Nor must you white knuckle through chaos alone. Every woman benefits exponentially leaning on diverse support - whether therapists, medical providers, friends, partners, coaches, family or community groups - for motivation setting health goals then encouragement achieving them. Shared experience breeds solidarity bolstering your tenacity.

This chapter explains different types of support to enlist easing uncertainty, validating complaints or reminding your worth when menopause knocks confidence. You need not traverse this winding road solo my friend! Let's build your village.

Who Provides What Support

Various members of your support squad will shine delivering specialized buckets of wisdom, practical advice or simply safe space to vent so you release bottled up emotions constructively versus spiraling down negative thought loops. Consider which needs you crave most right now:

Informational Support explaining menopausal changes and interventions comes from ob-gyns, registered dietitians, pharmacists, fitness pros, health coaches etc. People and resources educating you so confusion subsides.

Appraisal Support involves someone assessing your situation then affirming your feelings and self perception are valid. Therapists excel here along with insightful friends or mentors. Reduce self doubt!

Emotional Support encompasses compassionately listening, hugging it out or even crying together over struggles big and small so you feel heard, understood and cared for through challenges. Your people that "just get you" matter most dispensing non judgemental love.

Instrumental Support means tangible assistance - meal prep, childcare, pet duties etc - lightening loads off your overfilled plate so more bandwidth opens relaxing into self care. Spouses, family, neighbors or paid helpers contribute here.

Spiritual Support comes through things like prayer groups, meditation spaces, nature immersion or massage/bodywork invoking inner calm and renewing inspiration that menopausal unease shall pass. This breeds mental space and optimism.

While one or two individuals may provide a few support types, curating your diverse team ensures all basics get covered. Now let's outline specific members worth including for rounded support.

Build Your Dream Team

Below are key players you want ponying up encouragement, insight and assistance cheering your menopause marathon to the finish line!

Your Partner acts as quarterback calling plays from the front lines of your relationship supporting you daily. Hopefully they educate themselves about hormonal changes to extend extra empathy when you feel cranky, teary or tangled in sheets sweating from hot flashes.Communicate openly about needs.

Close Girlfriends that uplift and empower you serve as trusted cheerleaders through every life season but especially transitions with sex and relationship uncertainty. Lean into feminine circles boiling over with laughter, wisdom, nurturance and straight talk in safe space together.

Support Groups provide solidarity and tips without even needing to burden your inner circle venting the same complaints repeatedly. Local or online communities unite women at all menopausal stages. Facebook and MeetUp offer options to explore by geography or interest like fitness, sexuality, health etc.

Your Gynecologist gives medical guidance about symptom management, testing health markers like cholesterol and bone density for risk factors or discussing pros and cons of hormone therapy approaches. Track cycles, lifestyle changes and symptoms to identify patterns helping them evaluate and support you.

Registered Dietitians offer personalized nutrition advice catering to your health conditions, fitness goals and symptom struggles. Ditch guessing games on the latest fad diets for science backed solutions from those formally trained. Find ones specializing in women's health concerns for bonus expertise.

Mental Health Pros like counselors or psychologists help reframe perspective when menopausal frustrations, body image issues or managing stressful life circumstances simultaneously overwhelm coping reserves. Build emotional skillsets preventing temporary circumstances from cascading into anxiety or depression if mood disorders run in your family.

fitness trainers, health coaches and bodyworkers like yoga instructors, Pilates pros, massage therapists or osteopaths address physical discomforts like stiff joints, low energy and muscle loss guiding appropriate movement modifications, hands on assistance releasing built up tension and advice preventing injuries. Customize activities that energize you while also preventing declines in strength or mobility.

Build and lean into your diverse support crew strategically during menopausal years and beyond. Getting promoted to crone status with its associated wisdom and reverence reflects not isolation but intense backend work cultivating community able to share the load and speak truth boldly whenever crises arise on this lifelong journey of growth. You were never meant to figure out everything alone! Together we thrive.

Part III: Training & Fueling For Vitality

With science based understanding about menopause mechanisms established along with relief strategies easing temporary discomforts, let's shift gears optimizing fitness and nutrition support for achieving awesome health, body composition and performance decades beyond our fertile years.

Consider Part III your playbook for training and fueling strategically through the menopausal transition while also setting yourself up for ultra functionality pursuing second act goals for whatever vibrant adventures await.

We'll cover optimizing exercise and eating considering your changed endocrine environment including:

- Hormone aware training modifications

- Strength priorities that transform body composition

- Cardiovascular health optimization

- Injury prevention and recovery protocols

- Macronutrient needs through menopause

- Mitigating metabolism slow down

- Gut health and microbiome factors

- Collagen, adaptogens and supplements to support goals

With expertise guiding appropriate fitness and fueling strategies catered to your unique menopausal mile markers, frustrations subside and inspiration builds appreciating this complex dance. What diet or training approaches worked easily in your 20s or 30s no longer serve the same way with declining estrogen, body composition changes and lifestyle shifts. Play the long game leveraging science for adaptation across years - even decades - ahead.

Get ready to feel empowered by your body again instead of fighting inevitable changes! Beyond surviving you will thrive. Now let's dig in...

Exercise Guidelines for Perimenopause & Postmenopause

Let's dive right into optimizing fitness for supporting your best health and functionality through the winding menopausal road ahead.

While no woman escapes aging, strategic training adaptations matching your body's evolving needs as hormones shift can mean the difference between disability, fatigue and weight gain accelerating your decline versus continuing to kick ass in cardio classes feeling strong pushing grandkids on swings 30 years down the road. Mindset and methodology matter hugely influencing long term outcomes even amid unavoidable changes.

This chapter breaks down specifics on:

- Realistic mindset resets around aging and athletic performance

- Training methodology adjustments to prevent injury

- Appropriate workout programming tweaks

- Recovery and injury prevention protocols

- Sample weekly training template

My aim is equipping you to set appropriate expectations that honor your body's current capacity while also modifying variables fully within control keeping your chassis rolling smoothly for decades to come. You've got this! Now let's dig in.

Mindset Resets

Before detailing specific TRAINING program variables, we need a mindset check. Most women hit an identity crisis as fitness metrics like strength gains, pace times or endurance seemingly nose dive against our will during perimenopause and menopause thanks to unavoidable physiological changes.

A grieving process often ensues mourning our youthful abilities which erodes motivation continuing healthy movement at all at the same level. Expectations feel unrealistic now. "Why bother since I'll never PR again?" becomes justification slipping into inactivity and consequently accelerated physical decline.

Flip mindsets sabotaging your fitness potential 40+ years post menopause! Here's how:

1.**Acknowledge inevitabilities but reject worst case scenarios.** Your cardiovascular capacity and strength stats cannot defy aging's effects. However with consistent smart training you still demonstrate MUCH higher function decades older than sedentary peers. Don't falsely equate some performance downgrade to justifying full on quitting! Certainly 120 year olds don't break world records but they also don't sit immobilized without independence thanks to continual movement. Find reasonable expectations.

2.**Focus more on consistency than continual progression.** Can you maintain prior strength numbers or pace efforts rather than expecting linear gains forever? Even sustaining current benchmarks despite hormonal odds stacking against you proves impressive! Celebrate capability over comparison.

3.**Redefine metrics for success** as you age. Rather than fastest miles or most weight lifted highlight more qualitative metrics like minimizing joint pain during activity, avoiding sickness that keeps you from workouts all winter or hitting 80% planned sessions per month. Judge yourself against realistic standards.

Now equipped with healthier perspectives, let's examine what elements of training itself to modify protecting those realistic standards through years ahead.

Methodology Adjustments

Regarding broad framework for structuring workout weeks, consider these common sense tweaks:

- Sub out one higher intensity session for extra active recovery like yoga, walking or easy cycling weekly

- Shorten session duration slightly if hit by fatigue or losing focus

- Limit high impact, plyometric or extremely grinding sessions

- Practice active isolation stretching post-workouts to increase pliability

Listen closely each day for joint pains or low energy cues indicating when to pull back intensity, duration or training load in order to support recovery. Remain consistent showing up with 80% effort on days you feel blah still nets benefits long term over skipping workouts or not fueling properly.

Program Specifics Tweaks

Getting more precise with actual program design components, these modifications help avoid overuse injuries and stagnation:

- Build progression mostly through volume increases before intensity bumps

- Cycle harder training blocks of 2 weeks then 1 week active recovery

- Balance pressing strength work plenty of posterior chain focus

- Perform unilateral and single leg exercises reducing shear forces

- Try offset loading modalities like Pilates reformer or Gyrotonics

Emphasize strength and stability during the menopausal transition deprioritizing cardio dependent improvements. Support whatever aerobic activity keeps you consistent like walking or gentle swimming but without much worry over pace, distance or output declines inevitable as hormones shift.

Nutrition Support

You know the nutrition fundamentals already but during menopause doubly emphasize::

- Meet daily protein needs - up to 1 gram per pound of body weight - to prevent muscle wasting

- Load anti-inflammatory foods like wild caught fish, colorful produce, nuts and olive oil

- Properly fuel workouts; hydrate really well before, during and after sessions

- Take recovery seriously - sleep, meditation, massage, epsom salt baths etc

Don't allow hard training to go to waste paired with inadequate nutrition support. Monitor macro ratios to prevent protein or healthy fats lagging too far behind carbohydrate intake.

Mindset For Motivation

Finally, stay motivated through inevitable ebbs and flows using these psychological tips:

- Practice self-compassion on off days

- Focus on consistency over continual progression

- Define success via enjoyment vs objective metrics

- Surround yourself with community support

- Remind yourself change remains temporary

You've got this! Training during menopause and beyond pays dividends but best heed methodology, nutrition and mindset considerations empowering your next stage of fitness. Expect ups and downs while celebrating little breakthroughs like newfound mobility or those surprise strength PRs sneaking up on you suddenly even amidst hormonal chaos. Your strong capable body keeps pleasant surprises in store if you listen closely. Now let's see sample workouts and splits in action.

Sample Weekly Training Plan

Below is a balanced weekly schedule blending strength circuits, multi plane yoga, easy cardio intervals and targeted stretching to maintain overall fitness protecting your hormones, heart health, mobility and Happiness through menopause:

Monday - Lower Body Strength
3 sets x 8-15 reps each leg for: Bulgarian Split Squats, Sumo Deadlift, Side Lying Clamshells

Tuesday- HIIT Cardio 25 minutes moderate pacing alternating 1 minute harder efforts with 2 minutes easy

Wednesday- Upper Body Strength
3 sets x 8-12 reps each side for: Single Arm Row, Incline Chest Press, Shoulder Reverse Fly

Thursday- Restorative Yoga 45 minute class focused on hip openers, gentle backbends and meditation

Friday - Total Body Metabolic Circuit
3 rounds performing 30-60 seconds work followed by 30 seconds rest for: Skater Hops, Pushups, Squat Jumps, Planks

Saturday - Long Walk 60-90 minutes moderate pace outside

Sunday - Active Stretching & Foam Roll 30-45 minutes head to toe mobilities

This balances your major movement patterns and fitness domains while allowing appropriate rest and recovery for tissue adaptation. Structure training weeks smartly catering workouts to your changing body listening when more rest proves prudent!

Sample Workouts For Strength, Cardio & Flexibility

Now let's get specific planning sample workouts that build balanced strength protecting hormone sensitive areas like pelvis, hips and spine while maintaining joyful mobility through the moderate cardio and strategic stretching.

I'll provide detailed sequences across categories personalized to common menopausal vulnerabilities like bone density loss, muscle wasting metabolism declines and joint instability. You can plug these templates straight into your existing routine or mix and match building a whole customized training program.

We'll cover:

- Total body metabolic strength circuit

- Lower body mobility flow

- Posterior chain and posture yoga

- Bone density boosting lifting plan

- Low impact cardio pyramid

The goal is demonstrating creative ways to train across functional domains that specifically serve health and resilience during the menopausal transition without requiring fancy equipment or high intensity efforts. You've got this!

Metabolic Strength Circuit

This total body Wham, Bam style circuit blends compound strength moves with bursts of cardio driving up calorie burn and hormonal response in minimal time while preventing boredom.

Try this sequence 2-3 times through, performing each exercise for 40 seconds all out effort then 20 seconds rest before the next. Cool down stretching afterwards. That's it!

The full menu with video links:

Mountain Climbers- High knees explode up catching core on fire

Goblet Squat to Overhead Press- Strengthens legs, glutes and shoulders dynamically

Split Stance Single Arm Row- Unilateral pull engages back and legs individually

Lateral Shuffle to Balance- Agility challenges hips while improving coordination

Pushup to Rotational Chop- Pushes then pulls upper body through multiple angles and patterns

Sumo Squat Hold With Bicep Curl- Tests legs and arms isometrically burning out muscles

Plank Up Downs- Serious core and shoulder stability requisite

Modify intensity lowering or raising the load - whether using bodyweight, dumbbells or resistance bands. Catch your breath fully before repeating circuits. Let's hit lower body and hips next.

Lower Body & Hip Mobility Flow

Counter all that pressing and squatting work with targeted stretches opening tight hip flexors, outer glutes and hamstrings that wreak havoc on posture. This sequence also builds coordination branding new neural patterns.

Perform 5-8 reps of each exercise, holding end range stretches for 2 full breaths. Complete 1-3 circuits flows.

- Fire Hydrant circles

- Hip Hinge Touch Opposites

- World's Greatest Stretch

- Frog Pump

- Bow Pose

- Low Lunge With Back Knee Down

- Walking Pigeon Stretch

- Lizard Lunge

- Happy Baby Pose

- Supine Figure Four

While strength training protects existing muscle avoiding estates atrophy as metabolism downshifts from estrogen changes and aging, sufficient mobility work ensures you access strength freely without unnecessary strain or compensation. Let's hit key areas needing extra attention next.

Posterior Chain & Posture Yoga

The rounded modern lifestyle wreaks havoc on our neck, mid back mobility and glute medius strength resulting in common tightness, pain and soreness. This targeted yoga flow counteracts wasting along the posterior muscle chain.

Move slowly through 5-8 breaths each pose focusing on full exhales softening contracted areas:

- Child's Pose

- Downward Facing Dog

- Sphinx Pose

- Cobra Pose

- Low Lunge Variation With Back Knee Down

- Warrior One

- Extended Side Angle

- Half Moon

- Seated Spinal Twist

- Legs Up The Wall Pose

This sequence stretches calves and hamstrings, strengthens low back and opens hips, mid back and shoulders simultaneously - all crucial for maintaining mobile stability as we age. Now let's deliver key areas impacting bone mineral density next.

Bone Density Boosting Lifting

Right about the age estrogen production starts tapering in perimenopause, women begin losing bone density rapidly from imbalanced bone building cell activity. Strength training - especially using external load not just bodyweight-

potently signals for increased bone density protecting against osteopenia, fractures and poor calcium metabolism.

Aim to lift 3 days a week focusing on compound movements in good form. Perform 2-4 sets of 8ish repetitions using moderately heavy weights around 60-80% your 1 rep max if known. Regress loads when technique falters.

I recommend programming some combo of these bone builders each session:

- Goblet Squats

- Chest Press - Dumbbell Or Machine

- Hip Hinge Romanian Deadlifts

- Overhead Farmer Carry

- Pulldowns Or Assisted Pull-ups

- Step Ups

- Seated Rows - Cable Machine Or Bands

Additional supplemental exercises like lateral raises, bicep curls or tricep extensions boost results too by incorporating upper body pulling and pushing but maintain solid squat/hinge/carry/row foundations stimulating skeletal strength strategically during the menopausal window. Now let's cover cardio.

Low Impact Cardio Pyramid

While most women recognize consistently elevating heart rate through aerobic conditioning protects long term cardiovascular and metabolic health into elder years, many dread chronic joint pain flaring up from excess pounding.

Lower impact options like swimming, rowing machines or incline walking provide solutions!

I recommend building "intensity pyramids" where you gradually spike effort over 10-20 minutes then recede again to control levels for joint comfort, pacing respiration and redirecting blood flow.

For example a beginner pyramid on a recumbent bike:

- Min 1-3: Warm up easily

- Min 3-6: Moderate pace able to breath comfortably

- Min 6-8: Challenging resistance adding intensity

- Min 8-10: Hard pushing nearing maximal steady pace

- Min 10-15: Backing down gradually nearing moderate

- Min 15-20: Cool down lightly

You can apply this concept to any machine safely where joints remain supported or low impact modalities isolating legs like swimming hip driven strokes. Walking or running outdoors works too backing off surfaces for descending efforts.

Not only do cardiorespiratory pyramids provide a fun mental distraction maintaining progressively harder intervals, they optimize conditioning effects spurring metabolic adaptations and oxygen delivering capillary growth in active muscles without overstressing connective tissue too much. Win win!

Commit just 2-3 days weekly to steady state low impact cardio starting around 30 minutes building duration as able. Support these habits with sound nutrition we'll cover next fueling your fitness potential through menopausal transitions and far beyond! Consistency conquers.

Performance Nutrition After Menopause

With smart fitness programming dialed balancing strength, flexibility and cardio development across the seasons of fertility decline and beyond, what we eat proves equally pivotal fueling that active potential so hard work outs don't go to waste or get derailed by metabolic shifts or inflammation exacerbating common menopause symptoms.

Optimizing nutrition allows us to feel awesome everyday pursuing passions while also driving disease protection stemming unavoidable increased risk from estrogen loss. Think thriving not just surviving!

This chapter will cover nutrition specifics in areas of:

- Calorie Needs Changes

- Macronutrient Ratios

- Hydration Guidelines

- Mitigating Metabolism Slow Down

- Blood Sugar Regulation

- Gut & Inflammation Factors

- Nutrient Timing Around Exercise

My aim is painting a complete picture how proactive eating supports vitality physically and mentally during the menopausal transition and post fertility while also setting you up nicely for ultra functionality many decades beyond. Let's eat well to live fully!

Calorie Needs Dropping

We all notice metabolism slowing incrementally each year even following consistent healthy habits. Weight seems to creep up annually regardless. But the decline shifts into overdrive during the menopausal transition thanks diminishing muscle mass from aging plus hormone changes fanning metabolic flames.

You simply require less daily energy burn to maintain prior weight as you navigate perimenopause into post menopause - about 50-100 calories fewer each passing year. This means if you ate 2400 calories at 35 years old to feel good and hold stable pounds, dropping to 2200 or below proves prudent by 50.

Tracking trends through a consistent food journal helps identify caloric sweet spots minimizes need for extreme cuts provoking rebound binges later or sacrificing proper nutrition. Embrace the decrease as permission enjoying smaller satisfying meals!

Macronutrient Ratio Shifts

Beyond slightly decreasing total calories keeping pace with a slowing metabolism, reconsidering ratios of carbohydrates, proteins and fats also optimizes body composition, energy levels and symptom management during the menopausal transition.

Estrogen and progesterone changes disrupt once effortless blood sugar regulation and insulin effectiveness. Concurrently, aging muscle mass burns less glucose and calories at rest. Dietary protein and healthy fats balance the transition preventing energy crashes, destructive sugar spikes and emotional lows while supporting retained strength.

Here are optimal macro ranges to try:

- Protein - 20-30% daily calories

- Fats - 30-40% daily calories

- Carbohydrates - 40-50% daily calories

This divides up something akin to 1 gram protein per pound of body weight, ample plant fats like avocado or nuts and moderate whole food carbs keeping blood sugar balancing smoothly.

Hydration Needs

Another non negotiable for supporting health amidst declining hormones rests on adequately hydrating both day to day and peri-workout. Being even mildly dehydrated exacerbates temperature regulation issues like hot flashes and night sweats. Headaches happen more easily too.

Aim for the following:

- Daily intake - at least 2/3rd your body weight in fluid ounces

- Pre workout- 12-16 oz electrolyte beverage

- During sessions- 5-8 oz every 30 minutes

- Post training- 16-24 oz electrolyte/protein mix

Monitor urine color as an easy metric ensuring you drink enough to maintain light lemonade to clear colors throughout day indicating well hydrated kidneys. Dark yellow signals push more fluids, particularly in summer months.

Mitigating Metabolism Drops

You can absolutely counteract a lowered metabolism by supporting anabolic muscle building pathways and thus bigger calorie burning engines at rest through properly fueling exercise recovery. The three keys involve:

1.**Consuming 20-25 grams complete protein** (like Greek yogurt, eggs or a shake) within 30-60 minutes post training to supply amino acids to damaged muscle fibers right when cells demonstrate greatest uptake capacities for regeneration.

2.**Mixing creatine compounds** into your post workout meal or supplement routine since research confirms this muscle powerhouse both increases lean mass development AND prompts greater insulin sensitivity benefitting blood sugar management long term. 5 grams daily helps most females max out potential stores.

3.**Not fearing healthy fats pre or post training** because quality anti inflammatory omega fatty acids from salmon, avocados, nuts or MCT oils help buffer inflammation from demanding sessions but also fuel hormones like testosterone that otherwise diminish for women at menopause hampering strength and metabolic gains.

Supporting Blood Sugar Balance

Speaking of hormones intersecting with nutrient metabolism, optimizing blood sugar regulation through thoughtful carbohydrate management proves paramount for maintaining energy, focus and stable moods as estrogen declines. Glycogen storage and insulin effectiveness both depend partially on estrogen signaling so deficiencies leave you vulnerable to crashes, cravings and downstream adrenaline rollercoasters once beloved pasta or popcorn binges now backfire. Help yourself by:

1.**Choosing nutritious whole food carb sources full of fiber** - vegetables of all colors, legumes and beans, minimally processed whole grains like quinoa, some fruits like berries. These break down slower preventing dangerous spikes and crashes.

2.**Pairing carbs with protein, fat or both** every meal and snack to balance absorption for steadier insulin response and appetite signaling. Trying beans and avocado, sweet potato and eggs or yogurt with granola all work!

3.**Supplementing cinnamon, berberine, fiber blends and magnesium** which all research confirms assists healthy glycemic regulation and insulin functioning for women with metabolic challenges like those common at menopause.

4.**Exercising regularly** maintains insulin receptivity so cells more readily store carbs as glycogen and blood glucose clears quicker rather than overflowing to be stored as excess body fat worsening weight loss struggles.

The Microbiome Impact

Nowadays you've certainly heard buzz about "gut health" and importance of our microbiome - trillions of beneficial bacteria and yeasts living symbiotically in our digestive tracts. These microflora directly influence nutrient absorption capacity, inflammation regulation, immune function plus neurotransmitters like serotonin modulating brain issues like anxiety, depression and focus.

Supporting a robust, diverse microbiome prevents gut issues driving central weight gain/blood sugar dysregulation but also improves mental health struggles frequently exacerbated during the menopausal transition.

Here's how to optimize your internal digestive ecosystem:

1.**Eat ample produce daily** full of polyphenols and resistant starches that "feed" good bugs like Lactobacillus and Bifidobacterium species strengthening their numbers in the gut.

2.**Consume fermented foods** like unsweetened yogurt, kefir, kimchi, sauerkraut, kombucha introducing complementary microbes that take up residence in your community.

3.**Consider targeted supplements** including sporeforming strains like Bacillus subtilis or Saccharomyces Boulardii if you must take antibiotics or deal with chronic intestinal problems like reflux, constipation or irritable bowels.

4.**Avoid highly processed foods and unnecessary antibiotics** which damage delicate balance of microflora. Read labels to identify preservatives, emulsifiers and artificial sweeteners disrupting optimal diversity.

Remember, gut balance links directly to mental health and hormonal health so inconsistencies trigger systemic inflammation exacerbating common menopausal complaints! Eat more plants, ferments and fiber.

Nutrient Timing Around Exercise

Finally let's connect how properly fueling exercise itself - before, during and after workouts - makes or breaks your capacity actually benefiting from all that hard training rather than insufficient calories or poor food choices blunting potential fitness gains thanks to hormonal mismatches. Follow three simple fueling commandments:

1. Before - Eat easily digested carbs up to 3-4 hours pre training supplying muscles adequate glycogen storage. Example: banana with nut butter, oatmeal with berries, or toast with honey. Wash down with 12-16 oz electrolyte beverage finishing drink 30 minutes prior.

2. During - Sip electrolyte fluids like coconut water every 20-30 minutes to replace sweat losses. For longer sustained endurance sessions try honey sticks or whole food bites like raisins every 45 minutes.

3. After - Consume 15-25 grams complete protein like Greek yogurt, eggs, beef or a smoothie blended with collagen peptides within 30-60 minutes post training along with veggie carb sources like sweet potatoes. The anabolic window for tissue repair spans 0-2 hours post exercise. Don't miss it! Replenish electrolytes too.

Properly fueling around training requires planning habits in advance so you consistently support each session. Set yourself up for wins — then actually realize them through strategic nutrition all day every day. That "bikini body" for those hot flashes comes down to daily mindfulness more than extreme temps in gym. You've got this!

Supplements to Support Your Goals

Reaching menopause signals shifting nutritional needs to compensate for declining hormones, slowly decreasing energy requirements yet often increased cravings. Supporting daily micronutrient status through smart supplementation fills gaps ensuring your body works optimally as metabolism evolves.

Targeted supplements also counteract common symptoms like hot flashes or joint pain for improved quality of life in the short term. Further several compounds show early promise defending long term health though research continues unfolding for anti-aging candidates.

This chapter outlines science backed supplemental supports I recommend women consider adding through perimenopause, menopause and beyond aligned to priorities like:

- Relief from disruptive symptoms

- Guarding heart health & body composition

- Strengthening bones & mobility

- Sharpening cognition & mood

- Supporting sleep quality

- Boosting energy levels & immunity

Keep perspective that while strategic supplementation helps optimize wellbeing as you transition through menopausal stages, nutrients work synergistically with lifestyle pillars like nutrition, mindset and fitness habits covered previously. Let's unfold specifics!

Relieving Unpleasant Symptoms

If bothersome issues like hot flashes, night sweats or similar menopause discomforts continue interfering with normal function after implementing lifestyle remedies from earlier chapters, these compounds offer additional relief for many women:

Isoflavone Phytoestrogens from soy foods or supplements provide mild activity binding estrogen receptors and cooling hot flashes similar to low dose hormone therapy for some women. Meta analyses found between 30-50% frequency reduction taking 50-100mg isoflavones from soy, red clover or kudzu daily.

Black Cohosh also demonstrates modest hot flash relief benefit for about 1 in 2 women at Remifemin's studied dosage of 40mg black cohosh compounds twice daily. Its mechanisms remain unknown but may involve serotonin or inflammatory pathways.

Omega 3 Fish Oils making diet upgrades emphasizing fatty fish often calms night sweats and hot flash severity. If still unsatisfactory after a month also supplement combined EPA + DHA omega-3s dosed around 1000-2000mg daily.

Magnesium before bed soothes nervous system hyperactivity also reducing palpitations, anxiety and sleep disruption related with hot flashes for some women during sweaty nights. Take 300-450mg elemental magnesium from glycine, citrate or threonate forms.

Maca Powder shows early promise alleviating menopause symptoms like mood swings, low libido and energy dips in a few studies, but more research is still needed. Try 1,500-3000mg gelatinized maca.

Protecting Heart, Metabolic & Brain Health

The trio of cardiovascular, bone and cognitive health risks all rise as estrogen production wanes from menopause. Get ahead of potential threats using supplements as insurance:

Vitamin D3 reaching blood levels of 40-60 ng/mL protects both bone and heart health by regulating calcium absorption while also supporting neuromuscular coordination, immune function and inflammation pathways tied to chronic diseases. Take 1000-4000IU D3 daily scaling to your lab testing.

Omega 3 Fish Oils delivering anti-inflammatory EPA/DHA fats not only stabilize mood and hot flashes but also benefit cholesterol markers reducing plaque buildup in arteries lowering heart attack and stroke risks. Consume 1-2 grams daily.

B-Complex + Folate support energy pathways involved in metabolizing macronutrients while keeping homocysteine levels moderated decreasing dementia and heart disease risks as we age. Look for active/methylated forms like methylfolate, methylcobalamin etc.

Collagen Peptides supplying targeted amino acids declining with age promotes both skin elasticity and joint integrity. 10 grams daily improves wrinkles and mobility. Bone broth offers whole food collagen source too.

CoQ10 + PQQ represents potent mitochondrial energizers and antioxidants potentially staving aspects of physiological aging. 100-200mg daily helps cognitive function, egg quality and periodontal health.

Strengthening Mobility & Resilience

The trio of glucosamine, calcium and vitamin D3 and omega 3 fats work synergistically together preserving bone density and joint health as tissue integrity declines with lower estrogen levels after menopause:

Calcium & Vitamin D3 help slow bone loss turning over at accelerated rates once estrogen drops. 1200mg calcium split doses and 1000-4000IU vitamin D3 daily delivers protection.

Glucosamine + Chondroitin repair cartilage cushioning joint impact showing reduced knee pain and slower osteoarthritis progression at typical doses around 1500mg glucosamine sulfate plus 800-1200mg chondroitin daily.

Hyaluronic Acid injections restore viscosity to synovial fluid between joints increasing shock absorption and flexibility for 6 months at a time. Supplements show modest benefit.

Boosting Cognition, Memory & Focus

Support concentration plus working memory functions often declining through menopause using brain boosting compounds:

Bacopa Monnieri Ayurvedic adaptogenic herb upregulates neurotransmitter activity improving memory, anxiety and attention at 300mg daily dosing.

Ginkgo Biloba appearing promising for mild dementia also benefits cognitively intact adults combatting brain fog. Try

120-240mg standardized to 24% flavone glycosides and 6% terpene lactones.

Phosphatidylserine comprising 15% of all cell membrane phospholipids directly supports intercellular signaling, neurotransmitter production and glucose metabolism tied to clearer thinking. 100mg may assist memory and mood.

Lion's Mane Mushroom supplies bioactive compounds called hericenones and erinacines spurring nerve growth factor production which stimulates structural neural changes improving cognition. 500mg twice daily seems beneficial.

Deepening Sleep Quality

Prioritize nightly sleep consistency through menopause as foundational pillar optimizing all other health goals. If still not sleeping soundly after applying numerous sleep hygiene tactics from earlier chapter, compounds benefiting GABA activity, anxiety or pain often help:

Magnesium Glycinate or other chelated forms relax muscles while modulating neurochemistry involved with sleep onset. Take 200-400mg nightly.

L-Theanine is an amino acid in green tea boosting alpha waves deepening REM quality at 200mg before bed. Synergistic with magnesium.

CBD Oil modulates multiple neurotransmitter pathways reducing anxiety that disrupts rest. Start with 10-25mg nightly titrating up as needed.

Melatonin in very small 0.3-1mg doses restores circadian signaling without next day grogginess or hampering natural production long term.

5-HTP boosts serotonin converting to melatonin improving sleep quality without addictive properties when dosed 50-200mg nightly.

Don't underestimate prioritizing nightly sleep consistency through menopause as foundational pillar optimizing ALL other health goals! Make restfulness priority #1.

Boosting Immunity, Energy & Longevity

Finally a category of promising anti-aging candidates target supporting foundational wellness elements like energy production, stress resilience, and immune function deteriorating over longer time horizons:

NAD+ represents essential coenzyme for fueling mitochondrial ATP energy generation and hundreds of metabolic processes. Animal models show precursors nicotinamide riboside or nicotinamide mononucleotide (NMN) extend lifespan by 7-15% but human trials still ongoing.

Resveratrol functions as antioxidant found in red wine and grapes potentially slowing aging through epigenetic changes, DNA protection and inflammation reduction. 100-500mg long term supplementation seems reasonably beneficial.

Glutathione acts as your body's master antioxidant and liver detoxifier declining with age while also supporting immunity and mitochondria. Lipoceutical glutathione, NAC or milk thistle build stores.

Medicinal Mushrooms like cordyceps, reishi, chaga and turkey tail contain polysaccharides may enhancing immune cell production and regulation. Early evidence supports lowered cold and flu rates. 1,000mg combo daily.

While human trials remain limited proving anti-aging benefits from newer candidates like NAD+ precursors, results look very promising based on considerable rodent data! I encourage healthy women to cautiously experimentIQ under practitioner guidance after reviewing fundamentals like nutrition, lifestyle and basic supplementation.

Key Takeaways

And those are my top recommended supplements to consider through menopause specifically targeting relief from disruptive symptoms, fortifying foundational health pillars like bone density and cardiovascular protection in the short term plus emerging anti-aging prospects reducing inflammation and improving energy on the decades long timescale!

Remember your basic lifestyle habits like nutrition, sleep, stress management and exercise consistency form the true basis for supporting high level wellness and function. View targeted supplementation as "bonus insurance" fine tuning physiological processes optimally - not foundational to health alone. First refine broader habits and mindset, then enhance targeted areas needing more support via vitamins, minerals and nutrients working synergistically together.

Hopefully these evidenced based options provide starting points alleviating specific discomforts, improving micronutrient insurance, defending longer term health and possibly supporting longevity as you traverse the menopausal years and beyond feeling fantastic!

Part IV: Revitalizing Relationships & Pursuits

Bravo cultivating the self care skills, training adaptations and nutritional support covered so far to thrive through menopausal physical changes! Now let's level up beyond purely managing symptoms to truly elevating your relationships, purpose and passion entering this next stage.

While fertility and outrageous hormone fluctuations gradually stabilize after menopause, the opportunity opens for directing freed up mental bandwidth plus physical energy towards the deeply meaningful. Our wild ride becomes a blank canvass!

Maybe you finally complete that book drafted over years, return to postponed creative pursuits from college days or launch an inspired business concept. Or perhaps you pursue trips allowing immersive cultural or nature connection, dedicate time learning new hands-on skills like cooking elaborate feasts or gardening, focus volunteering to uplift community causes, enroll continuing education courses delving topics that fascinate or pour love into new grandchildren.

My intention through Part IV involves sparking ideas, addressing fears head on and equipping you with tactical tools setting the stage for relationship enrichment, engaging work, financial freedom, purpose alignment, passion projects or anything else your spirit longs to explore.

Menopause calms the physical intensity that dominated earlier life seasons making space to hear inner wisdom whisper, "What lights me up?" beyond previous roles and responsibilities. This clean slate allows redefining not just health habits but life trajectories from whole cloth without limitation. You direct this movie plot twist!

Maybe your purpose and community contributions crescendo volunteering with organizations you care about deeply. Or perhaps long subverted desires to grow artistic talents or make political/environmental impact emerge again ready for nurturance decades delayed. What calls the empowered wise woman within? Menopause frees us to courageously live out the answer.

Sometimes fears and excuses still interfere: crappy cultural messaging making women feel invisible, boring or useless post menopause. Outdated partner expectations stifling personal growth. Or false beliefs that vitality inevitably declines rendering goal pursuit futile.

LET'S OBLITERATE THOSE LIES starting now. Flip perspective recasting "common knowledge" on its head through these pages highlighting role models, paradigm shifters and everyday women thriving in passionate purpose post menopause instead of fading away. Catch the vision then make it yours!

Communicating with Partners About Changes

Navigating menopause while simultaneously keeping relationships happy and healthy amidst chaos often feels overwhelming! Declining hormones impact moods, sleep and libido feeding cycles jeopardizing harmony if unaddressed. Meanwhile cultural taboos prevent transparent conversations to head off downstream turmoil after misunderstandings brew resentment over time left unsaid.

This chapter provides straight talk equipping partners better support one another through transitional relationship rough patches and beyond. I offer tips setting positive foundations, unpack specific communication sticking points like flagging sex drives or hot flash annoyances and encourage boldly envisioning relationship ideals centered around compassion.

My hope is increasing mutual understanding about the psychological and physiological root causes behind common menopausal struggles so both individuals feel seen while also choosing patience and grace receiving imperfect support some days. Nurturing true intimacy, care and growth mindsets pave the way.

Communicating About Menopause

Open vulnerable dialogue remains foundational for maintaining emotional and physical connection through any long term relationship yet too often breaks down during seasons of change instead of deepening bonds. Solid partnerships require nurturance. Don't assume your partner "should" already know your needs and frustrations or vice versa without spelling specifics out clearly and often.

I encourage women wholeheartedly to become expert communicators about menopause experiences that men genuinely can't fully grasp. Share feelings freely then also suggest constructive ideas better fostering your flourishing rather than suffering silently, making subtle digs when disappointment boils over or downplaying very real impacts from biological shifts.

Likewise partners demonstrate investment loving well through compassionate curiosity, insight seeking and emotional presence instead of quick fixes when women confide menopause related struggles big and small. Ditch assumptions forged in ignorance or indifference. Move together with empathy centering her thriving.

This chapter offers realistic foundations, critical talking points and vision casting for rediscovering intimacy and care while releasing unrealistic expectations. Thriving partnerships in this season start with radical candor and unconditional listening on both sides. Are you ready? Let's begin...

Start With Compassionate Mindsets

Before addressing specific friction points like sexual disconnects or symptoms disrupting joint happiness, first establish shared value for compassion and self responsibility in relationships by asking yourselves:

1. Do we both lead assuming best intentions from one another or jump towards blame if support feels imperfect at times? Can we offer grace while also vulnerably sharing experiences and requests?

2. Are we willing to take ownership for individual wellbeing and fulfillment by voicing needs proactively

versus expecting a partner's actions to determine happiness?

3. How might stress or emotional baggage from other life domains unconsciously negatively impact our patience and perceptions within the intimate relationship if not addressed?

Instill the wise mindset upfront in your partnership that no one gets relationships perfectly "right" by default at every season - we all must commit to lifelong intention, effort and growth transcending biology. Define true love as an action verb together! With common vision established and pride set aside, identifying core frustrations becomes so much easier.

Key Talking Points

Below find the most frequent unspoken menopause related contention points cited by women as hurting intimate connections:

Declining Libido & Changing Sexuality

Shifting hormones like plunging testosterone coupled with vaginal discomfort drastically alter many women's arousal while they also wrestle body image and identity shifts from aging. Be honest communicating transformed sensual interests plus surprising new erogenous zones when old favorites lose intensity. Explore together patiently rather than ignoring changes. Solutions exist ranging from lubricants and hormones to pillow talk dispersing shame!

Physical Symptoms Disrupting Couple Life

Of course hot flashes, night sweats and bladder urgency disrupt daily routines let alone intimacy. Proactively warn partners what to possibly expect so odd behaviors make sense later. Way less weird to mention night sweats may hit beforehand if it helps normalize having sex with sheets drenched later or taking an abrupt cold shower when hot flashes strike while cuddling up watching movies. Give insight and humor releasing tension.

Increased Emotional Reactivity & Anxiety

If estrogen shifts predispose you towards feeling extra sensitive some weeks, speak up when heightened irritation, sadness or impatience bubble up faster than usual. Verify if intense reactions fit the facts of benign situations accurately or might partially stem from wonky hormones magnifying inner noise disproportionately. When self aware in moments, deliberately choose to exhibit gentler behaviors until passing rather than unleash overreactions inappropriately upon loved ones later feeling remorseful. Protect harmony proactively since menopause bears no blame.

Feeling Undesirable & Unsexy From Aging

Insecurities often torment women internally as metabolism slows, weight redistributes and signs of aging appear despite cultural conditioning falsely tying beauty and worth tightly together for feminine identity. Yet negative self talk couldn't stray further from the truth! Verbally reassure her while focusing attentively on attractive traits as partners gain deeper understanding - women's beauty and life phase appeal evolves rather than diminishes over decades for the wise. Reinforce that truth through genuine compliments, displayed desire and positive body language in her presence.

General Forgetfulness & Mental Fatigue

If loved ones seem more scatterbrained and less focused than usual for awhile, assume optimistically it indicates nothing about priorities and cut frustrated reactions. Neurological changes during the menopausal transition impair memory, concentration, multitasking and mood regulation temporarily but the situation improves in time. In the meantime, approach absent mindedness and distraction with compassion not judgment. Double check perceptions before reacting during phases partners seem "checked out" emotionally.

Pinpointing the most frequent "unspoken" areas of disconnect allows couples to preemptively normalize challenges and start important dialogue bridging gaps. No need to dread changes as though relational threats - instead bring them into light! Now let's envision ideals.

Reimagine Your Relationship Vision

Rather than just surviving rocky adjustment periods, use the menopausal transition as opportunity taking your long term partnership to whole new levels of mutual fulfillment by asking "What do we want for ourselves and this relationship looking ahead years and decades down the road?"

Dream together - then communicate desires through daily actions anchored to that North Star vision keeping sight on what matters most for "us" versus pettiness tempting couples off track temporarily.

Perhaps you visualize perfect comfort cultivated between one another - that partners remain ultimate safe space for raw honesty, wholehearted vulnerability and unconditional listening without judgement as bodies change, dreams evolve or insecurities surface.

Or you commit to nurturing intimacy through difficulty by persevering to understand needs plus foster trust and loyalty despite seasons that intimacy models must adapt because of hormone changes. Healing awaits for those brave enough to pioneer new patterns.

Maybe you pursue greater passion purposefully seeking out new ways for frequently connecting souls, discovering adventures together or dedicating yourselves to mutual growth chasing horizons beyond stale status quos.

Use this transition as catalyst for rediscovering the love, compassion and friendship that first bonded your hearts before the chaos of midlife or monotony of routine quashed your vibrant romantic spark over years. You choose the vision while also communicating pitfalls threatening your ideal relationship state.

Approaching external or internal menopause triggered friction as opportunities for intentional progress together rather than irrecoverable threats set your partnership on course thriving for decades vs tentatively just persevering. But first you must embrace candid communication and radical self responsibility. Dare greatly shaping the relationship you want!

Cultivating Intimacy & Satisfaction

Navigating changing hormones, aging bodies and decades of history together can undoubtedly complicate intimacy through midlife. Yet the menopausal transition also offers a bridge to profoundly deepening connection in partnerships for those bold enough to pioneer new models centered around authenticity, empathy and mutual nurturing.

Rather than settling for adequate or unfulfilling sex due to discomforts or assumptions that passion inevitably fades with age, I encourage you to shatter status quos and write a new story governed by courage not fear. This chapter lights the way with science-backed insights, tangible communication tools and inspiration from those discovering greater satisfaction through intention, prioritization and practice.

Redefining Intimacy

Before addressing physical intimacy specifically, let's expand limiting mainstream definitions of connection often hyperfocused on frequency of intercourse and orgasms. Beyond sex, true intimacy encompasses emotional and spiritual bonds cultivated through:

- Shared rituals fostering trust, care, joy

- Reciprocal nurturing inspiring growth

- Celebrating milestones big and small

- Overcoming adversity together

- Communicating openly and vulnerably

- Gazing into one another's souls

- Exploring new adventures side by side

- Creating something meaningful together

- Laughing hysterically until it hurts

My point being that intimacy lives not exclusively below the beltline but through everyday actions and presence. Start from a foundation of friendship, make deposits regularly emotional bank accounts and the "spark" organically follows.

Managing Physical Discomforts

Alright now onto dealing with menopause related struggles making consistent satisfying sex frustrating like vaginal dryness or vulvar pain interfering with arousal and penetration or hot flashes disrupting the moment.

First know you aren't alone - over half of menopausal women deal with pain, low libido or discomfort changing what enjoyment previously looked like. Yet practical solutions exist from lubricants to hormone therapy. Talk with your gynecologist tailoring relief to your symptoms and preferences.

Beyond treating issues, prioritize sexual wellness proactively through self care: continue exercising for blood flow, stay hydrated, manage stress and sleep deprivation, eat nourishing foods and carve out couple time for non-sexual touch like massage. Setting the stage for satisfaction requires planning not luck!

Bridging Desire Gaps

Another intimacy issue involves mismatched libidos through midlife with testosterone dropping for women yet remaining stable for most men. Understanding this hormonal change along with other biological differences around arousal can prevent taking perceived personal rejection so seriously.

Be patient with one another's transitions. Seek compromise meeting in the middle - maybe sexual frequency or initiation drops but you grow new aspects like sensual touch, playfulness or emotional connection. Recognize that flame still smolders inside even if expressing desire differently now.

Proactively share positive feelings and appreciation to foster receptivity while also becoming curious about new erogenous zones emerging. Prioritization and practice can reignite satisfying sex lives together again with this simple blueprint.

Talking Through Taboos

Of course open vulnerable communication remains foundational for overcoming friction points or changes in the bedroom. Yet discussing intimacy often stays shrouded in shame or secrecy given cultural taboos and gender socialization.

I encourage partners consciously creating safe space for radical truth telling - express insecurities, confess embarrassing struggles, voice formerly unmentionable desires without fear of judgement. And listen with empathy remembering change remains constant in long term relationships.

Questions to honestly ask one another might include:

- What currently satisfies or dissatisfies me sexually?

- What enjoyable activities could we try or bring back?

- How have my interests changed throughout phases of life, parenthood, aging?

- What inhibitions or assumptions limit my/our enjoyment and expression?

- How do I define all aspects intimacy beyond just intercourse?

- What makes me feel most connected emotionally and spiritually?

Keep discussing awkward topics openly without blame for the win together long term. Unaddressed disconnects or shame corrode relationships slowly over time. But courage and vulnerability metabolize threats into growth progressing partnership to deeper planes.

Inspiring New Possibilities Beyond 50

Rather than accepting cultural ageist nonsense about waning passion being inevitable, I encourage you to embrace midlife intimacy as an opportunity consciously evolving sexual relating to profoundly serve your souls through:

- Offering your full embodied authentic presence

- Savoring sensory pleasures free from goal oriented focus

- Exploring meaningful erotic touch beyond preconceived limitations

- Gazing adoringly into one another's eyes

- Bursting into laughter and playfulness

- Lovingly caretaking each other's needs

- Allowing time and space for awakened arousal

- Communing skin to skin heart to heart

- Moving together slowly with full body reverence

- Shamelessly vocalizing pleasure and desire

Beyond mechanics, discuss what emotional states and environments inspire feeling safe, relaxed, valued and adored facilitating satisfying encounters. Discover how intimacy shifts serving your growth and connection now compared to earlier parenting years. Then commit practicing that vision.

While menopausal hormone changes can complicate consistency, know that many women report their most emotionally fulfilling sex unfolding after 50 without the pressure or impatience of youth. Patience and creativity coupled with prioritizing time together lights enduring fire. Fan yours by courageously pioneering new patterns that set your relationship thriving for years ahead!

Following Your Passions & Purpose

The menopausal transition offers a pivotal moment taking stock of limiting beliefs, relationships or situations no longer serving your highest potential so you can realign towards passionate purpose again. Consider this time a catalyzing bridge to your next epic life chapter!

While earlier decades focused on building careers, raising families or accumulating stability, something shifts for many women as childbearing years wane. The external noise quieting down allows finally hearing an inner call to meaning unearthing buried dreams and talents.

Maybe you feel the pull towards leadership, activism or legacy building volunteering for causes close to your heart. Or perhaps latent creative talents or the drive towards connection now demand nurturance delayed for years tamped down by prior demands. What whispers await your listening now?

I encourage you to embrace midlife as opportunity ruthlessly shedding roles, routines or relationships keeping you small to courageously embody the leader, creator, explorer, visionary, nurturer, adventurer, catalyst, teacher, builder or healer you were destined becoming all along. This chapter lights the way!

Envisioning Your Next Horizon

Start by getting quiet envisioning how you want this next chapter unfolding - what brings vibrancy, meaning and adventure? Dream without constraint about impact pursing and talents developing.

What goals left unstarted tug your spirit—write that book, launch a coaching business, traverse exotic locales, run for office, create magnificent gardens? Which people or communities call you contributing sweat and soul?

Which passions or use of your gifts deliver such joy you lose track of time immersed? What environments make you feel most alive - academia, stages, boardrooms, forests, kitchens? The pen awaits your writing.

Overcoming Fears & Mental Blocks

Of course expired dreams and stifled talents stir resistance too - maybe you feel too old changing course or fear failure, finances or your family's reactions. Cultural nonsense insists women disappear quietly after 50.

Let's tear down those false narratives now with perspective and planning. Too old? Ridiculous. The average life expectancy stretches 40+ more years with peak cognition lasting decades not years. That leaves tons of runway fully becoming.

As for failure, f$&@ it! Fortune favors the bold and growth depends on missteps. Even "unsafe" career pivots appear less daunting after developing resilience and skillsets over decades of experience. Financial security through purpose trumps golden handcuffs.

Lastly if unsupportive relationships threaten your growth, compassionately seek alignment through dialogue or distance. You teach people how to treat you by modeling priorities unapologetically. Consider whether playing it safe avoiding discomfort benefits anyone long run. Probably not.

Now to shift from possibility to tangible planning...

Making It Happen

After identifying inspiring goals, break undertakings into stepwise processes balancing enlivening work alongside playfulness. Movement towards milestones keeps passion flowing flexible adapting plans as you learn.

Maybe volunteer projects unite friends sharing talents serving vulnerable groups before envisioning nonprofit spinoffs formalizing over years. Or perhaps night classes learning creative skills scratch subverted itches between corporate jobs eventually enabling entrepreneur side hustles taking flight.

Give space trying new personas beyond longstanding roles. Write terrible first drafts growing writing muscles without judging imperfect starts. Dabble freely surrendering perfectionist pressures that paralyze potential. Show up consistently chipping away resistance.

Not sure how to begin? Use these less overwhelming idea starters discovering what lights you up along the way:

- **Take Inventory:** What latent talents, life experiences or knowledge bases prime you for making a difference somehow? Teaching, writing, creating, humor, leading, connecting, advising, building, healing?

- **Tap Networks:** Who already surrounds you offering guidance towards purpose like mentors, colleagues, groups aligned in values? Consult their journey steps.

- **Learn Something New:** What topic areas fascinate like languages, spirituality, finance, cultures, activism, ecology? Indulge curiosity through classes, books or documentary binges noticing what hooks your intrigue during free time.

- **Revisit Old Dreams:** What posters decorated teenage bedroom walls envisioning someday selves - Travel? Perform music? Open bakeries? Ranch horses? Draw comics? Invent new technologies? Reignite embers abandoned long ago.

- **Switch Up Routines:** Boring days numb creativity and motivation reinforcing stuckness. Shake habits interviewing innovators, exploring new neighborhoods, changing playlists to ignite fresh ideas.

- **Do Things That Scare You:** Fear warns of aliveness. Lean towards emotional edges and self doubt. Let adrenaline beckon adventure.

Awakening purpose requires patient mining of soul layers too long ignored. Sift reflection and experimentation without demanding instant clarity or profitability. Trust emergence. Each small step strengthens courage, resources and community to support bigger leaps in time.

The motivated midlife woman holds immense power catalyzing her circumstances and the greater world. Now go wisely wield yours!

Embracing Your Sensuality

While mainstream messaging hyperfocuses menopausal sensuality on libido changes tied to intimacy with partners, I encourage you towards a more expansive empowering definition appreciating your sensual energy as women fully inhabiting our power at this life stage.

Consider sensuality the vital lifeforce pulsing through your every cell inviting aliveness through self expression, embodiment, pleasure and connection. Beyond sex, igniting your sensuality fuels creativity, confidence, inspiration and a more vibrant experience of living fully through all your days.

Igniting sensuality harnesses feminine magnetic energy traditionally celebrated in goddess traditions now modernized into everyday inspiration through movement, adornment, touch, and sisterhood.

This chapter offers ideas and practices helping you glow up hidden potency as a midlife woman through:

- Adorning your body proudly

- Moving in flow state freedom

- Indulging your senses

- Connecting through touch

- Surrounding in sisterhood

On Beautifying For Your Own Gaze

Begin by taking inventory of pieces adorning your body like jewelry passed down generations, tattoos symbolizing growth, or clothing honouring heritage and style. Do beloved items sit unworn resigned only for special occasions out of habit?

I encourage dusting off view-obscuring emotional cobwebs treat mementos as soul armor for daily life not just collecting dust. Wear meaningful bracelets, earrings or necklaces as talismans infusing confidence to overcome inertia. Display tattoos or piercings unapologetically despite cultural norms insisting on erasing older women's individualism and bodily autonomy.

Style your waist, decolletage, wrist, ankle, neck, ears or anywhere striking your fancy because midlife's too short denying self decoration bringing joy! This invitation to freely adorn your physical form serves as metaphor for proudly taking up space exactly as you are.

On Moving To Ignite Aliveness

Next channel vitality through movement honoring innate rhythms and pleasure. Dance freely with music channeling ancient goddesses pulsing regenerative life force energies.

Twirl carefree embracing your inner child's body wonder decades before critiques warped self perception. Let limbs cut loose through space unstiffened by cares as breath propels supple joints.

To dive deeper into danced embodiment beyond fleeting moments, explore classes like ecstatic dance, 5 rhythms or even striptease cardio tuning into poetry your hips and shoulders sing untethered by worries an audience might judge imperfect technique.

Who says only 20-somethings deserve experiencing unadulterated body joy through movement? Woman up with playful practices that leave you flushed and alive. Sensuality awaits unleashed through liberating steps.

On Indulging Your Senses For Immersion

Sensuality also lives through immersing your whole being - mind, body and spirit - into favorite sensory experiences like these:

- Let music saturate cells until chills run down spine moved to core by beloved songs. Sob out heartbreak ballads. Belt out power anthems roaring from bellies. Chant along mantras echoing ancestral medicine. Allow rhythm physically exorcise stuck trauma energy stored decades in tight muscles and fascia.

- Inhale extra slowly perfuming worlds bottled into essential oils. Anoint pulse points inviting memories linked to signature scents over years. Lavender soothes anxiety. Bergamot lifts gloom. Jasmine ignites courage. Tree resins ground spiritual connection. Take stock what emotional and physiological power notes unleash for you.

- Sink teeth into ripe juicy persimmons, succulent meats or favorite childhood candies. Massage oil droplets around tongue not rushing satiation. Allow morsels saturate senses unhurried relishing flavor profiles that make you swoon. Culinary nourishment deserves moved reverence.

Lean into favorite sensory gateways beyond rational mindfulness towards hedonistic immersion. What delights elicit your being's full body soul smile when given permission receiving without distraction or dilution? More awaits discovered.

On Touching To Transmit & Receive Energy

As women, our hands inherently hold healing, magic and feminine power transmitting wisdom, empathy, vitality, safety and unconditional positive regard through skin-to-skin connection. Yet many of us become touch deprived entering midlife single or disconnected from past roles like hands-on parenting young children.

Combat isolation and anxiety by proactively gifting therapeutically restorative touch through modalities like reiki, massage or reflexology swirling positive energies to yourself then paying forward comforting contact within community.

Sensuality lives through human hands - not just partners but also platonic friends, children, elders, sisters. Never hesitate reaching for sacred touch flowing from the divine feminine impulse to nourish. Our gentle strokes heal near instantly energy otherwise requiring years processing through words or tears.

On Activating "Sisterhoods"

Finally connect through feminine circles and communities multiplying collective sensual power. Covens and temples through the ages convened wise woman transmitting teachings and medicines forward grounded in trust, mentorship and solidarity politics. Network your modern "sisterhoods" too.

Among women you resonate with at soul level, let down survival guarding erected against daily gendered microaggressions and dangers. Stare proudly into mirrors of one another's eyes seeing perfect beauty reflecting back. Voice private pains or dreams only sisters can fully empathize through lived experience.

Ask sisters to gently cradle heaviness accumulated carrying unrealistic superwoman expectations. Request soft hands on shoulders bolstering when others misunderstand complex situations. Seek wisdom only decades living across diverse intersectional walks provides.

Within safe feminine sanctuaries made microcosms, ticklish joy surfaces aired casually in ways rarely possible amidst mixed company without ridicule risk. Giggles erupt louder, hair flips fly sassier and gentle teasing sticks words precisely where most needed hearing. Help sisters glow up.

Awaken personal sensuality then harness magical catalyzing properties uniting women's complementary essence. Your vital embodiment and empowerment multiplies rippling inspiration outward through communities. Now ignite!

Financial Planning for Midlife

While menopause itself may not directly impact your net worth, midlife remains a pivotal season financially as earlier career earnings peak, retirement decisions loom and priorities often pivot towards legacy building or enjoying hard won freedoms.

Whether tomorrow feels blank slate full of inspiring possibilities or anxiety inducing depending on savings accrued so far, purposeful planning ensures you can fund this next chapter aligned to evolving dreams rather than defaulting reactive mode.

This chapter provides an overview equipping you optimizing spending, protecting assets and maximizing investing literacy so money lubricates possibilities without limiting bold moves impacting purpose or passion projects ahead.

We'll tackle building wealth through midlife by:

- Getting clear on financial priorities

- Making spending align values

- Securing protections for health & longevity

- Investing 101 and retirement accounts

- Passive income streams & side hustles

- Estate planning and legacy goals

While finances feel boring to some, nothing proves more liberating than harnessing the power of money multiplying good through causes and communities you care about. Think

abundance flows. Read on to ensure you can fund dreams decades ahead!

Envisioning Purposeful Spending

Start financial planning exercises identifying your most meaningful lifetime goals then working backwards calculating required runways. Do soul searching vision exercises uncovering how pursuing purpose might necessitate funding education, launching businesses, supporting causes, lifting others through mentorship or whatever else your spirit longs leaving legacy.

Maybe performing music, developing inventions to progress society or pouring sweat equity into volunteer work matters most exceeding pure profit motives. Or perhaps dreams of extensive travel, language immersion or passionate projects finally receive focus after years devoted to high demanding careers or intensive parenting roles.

Either way, allocate earnings towards priorities resonating deepest in this season while eliminating lifestyle inflation or keeping up with Joneses in areas falling lower on values hierarchies. Times ahead promise freedom directing finances towards meaning making if wisely stewarded now.

Budgeting Values Based 'Buckets'

One helpful hack budgeting limited resources across competing priorities entails dividing spending categories into percentages like:

Needs

- Housing

- Utilities

- Insurance

- Debt

- Groceries

- Transport

True Happiness

- Fitness & Health

- Education

- Travel

- Passions

- Gifts/Donations

- Experiences

Nice Extras

- Dining Out

- memberships

- Clothing

- Technology

- Decor

Track outlays across recent months assessing how current habits serve your best life. Make incremental monthly tweaks if needed reducing extras diverting towards funding the meaningful matters stack. Mastering financial foundations frees pursuing purpose away from scarcity or fear!

Securing Health & Longevity

Of course preparing for decades beyond fertility means analyzing risks threatening independence or longevity like illness, accidents and end of life considerations also requiring safety net planning through appropriate insurances for needs spanning:

Health: Ensure coverage encompassing routine preventative, unexpected emergencies plus any chronic issues already under management with access to your trusted providers. Catching problems early saves.

Disability: If injured or facing health situations potentially impacting work capacity short or long term, disability coverage provides part salary replacement so you can focus fully on healing without compounding money stressors.

LongTerm Care: With average life expectancy stretching years beyond previous norms, evaluate needs and options funding full time care if unable assistance completing regular daily living activities alone given certain age related decline.

Estate Planning: More on this below but get ducks in row designating healthcare power of attorneys, living wills, estate executors and other legal protections guaranteeing your wishes and legacy intentions are carried out in event of incapacitation or death. Plan for longevity!

While slightly uncomfortable proactively peering into worst case scenarios, being prepared allows sleeping easier and focusing present moments more fully knowing that health and wealth feel protected regardless of whatever unknowns life brings.

Retirement Investing 101

Retirement savings often fall short given the realities of disrupted careers, pay inequity or prioritizing family needs over consistent contributions yet hope persists catching up. Luckily time remains on your side with the right strategies taught never too late by financial educators.

Here's an overview if new approaching investing potentially supplementing social security or tying over between endeavors:

Retirement Vehicles: Beyond savings accounts, most tax advantaged retirement plans falls into two categories—defined contribution like 401Ks where you choose investments or defined benefit pensions with set monthly payouts afterwards. Know options.

Tax Advantages: Certain accounts offer incentivized savings through pre-tax contributions, tax deferred growth and preferential tax treatment upon withdrawal. Learn rules maximizing benefits for your situation like deductible IRAs.

Employer plans: If your workplace offers retirement accounts like 401Ks with possible matching incentives, always contribute minimums guaranteeing you don't leave free money on table.

Investing Basics: Seek help selecting appropriate asset allocation between stocks, bonds etc balancing reasonable risk and returns aiming for at least 8% yearly through compounding over decades.

Even starting modestly today leveraging tax advantages and employer incentives pays exponential dividends over long run. Avoid paralysis overwhelmed by options. Start somewhere charting course corrections needed.

Passive Income & Side Hustles

Another smart strategy diversifying income streams involve creating supplementary revenue pipelines needing less active hours from you directly through avenues like:

Passive Income: Assets earning money while you sleep like owning real estate collecting rents or investing royalties from intellectual property like books, courses or products created and sold online

Side Hustles: Monetizing existing assets intermittently like renting living space through home shares, hosting virtual experiences tied to your skills, leading specialized workshops or selling crafts/products you create

Building passive income or tapping side hustles provides flexibility earning beyond typical hourly means allowing more freedom pivoting careers paths, reducing workload stresses or saving towards legacy dreams on your timeline not dictated by monthly paychecks alone.

And remember extra income allows greater generosity making positive difference through causes aligning deepest values feeding souls too. Uplevel smartly.

Estate Planning For Legacy

Lastly but most important rests planning for assets distribution intentionally carrying forward your legacy with heirs and causes closest resonating with identity beyond this lifetime. Estate planning remains vastly complex and personal process but here are key considerations:

Beneficiaries: Name who exactly receives assets from retirement accounts, insurance payouts and properties ensuring fairness aligning values if disputes arise between blended families.

Trusts: Establish legal transfer processes protecting inheritance assets until beneficiaries reach appropriate ages managing sums responsibly themselves such as minors inheriting money intended later education uses

Wills: Spell exactly what assets gets left to whom in event of incapacitation or death appointing trusted executors enacting final wishes avoiding court decisions by default

Charitable Donations: Fund causes changing lives meaningfully through donor advised funds gifting during life then carried over through estate dollars making multiplying positive impacts into the future

Advanced Directives: Prevent medical wishes being disregarded unable speaking for self by preemptively documenting exactly which life preserving measures you want or don't want applied if facing terminal diagnoses or permanent unconsciousness then legally naming someone advocating on your behalf. Alleviate future burdens upon loved ones struggling guessing amidst grief and discord about what aligns your personal ethics and quality of life preferences if unable actively directing your care plan yourself one day. Better clear now!

While seizing midlife for pursuing passion fills coming days with meaning and aliveness, responsible planning ensures you can also direct hard earned money towards whatever matters most financially for people or charities later too. Seek trusted guidance sorting multi-pronged options matching hopes. Fund your purpose then purposefully fund heirs to pay it forward.

Part V: Your Action Plan

We've covered immense ground so far addressing everything from menopausal physiology, symptom relief hacks and fitness strategies to relationship communication tools, financial planning, passion project ideas and more. Now emerges the active application phase putting insights into practice!

Consider Part V your launching pad solidifying key lessons learned into customized action plans for elevating health, happiness and purpose day-to-day through perimenopause, menopause and beyond.

I'll provide goal setting worksheets helping you nail down specific wellness targets and metrics keeping momentum. You'll find troubleshooting tips when inevitable obstacles arise so you pivot back on track again. We'll cover:

- Crafting Your Inspiring Vision

- Defining Needs & Setting Goals

- Tracking Metrics that Motivate

- Accountability Hacks

- Rewriting Limiting Belief Stories

- Celebrating Mini Wins

Ultimately you determine how to harness menopause as catalyst claiming expanded vitality and purpose or just maintaining status quo. I offer the playbook but you call plays manifesting reality through courageously embodying the leader, lover, creator, explorer, visionary, healer and vibrant wise woman already inside.

Think captaining sports teams pre gaming the championship. Coaches sketch Xs and Os but players must execute with excellence. We'll map your playbook then cheer bold follow through!

Keep what serves from earlier sections: hormone balancing tactics easing physical discomfort, stress busting rituals supporting mental health, improved nutrition and movement patterns serving fitness, financial strategies multiplying freedom. Then build upon strong foundations personalizing tools setting you up thriving continuously, not just coping when crises hit.

Your phase of life sets up impact rippling into society and future generations more exponentially than ever through guidance, grit, emotional intelligence, spiritual connectivity, passion projects and legacy building. But first do the inner work sculpting resilient mindset and consciously directed days. Sweat the small stuff transforming thoughts and habits so big picture dreams unfold.

I can't wait to hear where implementing your menopause playbook takes you 5, 10, 20+ years ahead. This transitional gateway promises not an ending but rather your chance finally authoring a beginning completely aligned with your truest soul. Write the story only you can live then boldly become it! The world needs your empowered wise woman leadership now more than ever. Are you ready to claim your calling? Let's get going!

Pulling It All Together

We've covered immense ground exploring everything from menopausal physiology, symptom relief hacks and fitness strategies to relationship tools, financial planning, purpose alignment and more. Now it's time to pull insights together into customized action plans elevating your daily health, happiness and empowerment through perimenopause, menopause and beyond!

Consider this chapter the launchpad solidifying lessons learned into reality through courageous next steps. I'll provide tactical goal setting guides, tracking metrics that motivate and troubleshooting advice so you manifest tangible progress. We'll tackle:

- Crafting an Inspiring Vision

- Defining Needs & Setting Goals

- Tracking Metrics that Motivate

- Rewriting Limiting Belief Stories

- Accountability Hacks

- Celebrating Mini Wins

Ultimately you determine how to harness menopause as catalyst claiming expanded vitality and purpose or just maintaining status quo. I offer the playbook but you call plays through embodying the leader, lover, creator, explorer, visionary, healer and vibrant wise woman already inside.

Think how championship sports teams apply coaching strategies to successful outcomes. We'll map your playbook then cheer bold follow through!

Crafting an Inspiring Vision

Sustaining motivation long term requires igniting inspiration and meaningfully improving daily experience not just achieving arbitrary targets. Outcome goals lacking connective tissue to personal values wither on vines when discipline fades.

That's why we start crafting an elevated vision for this stage of womanhood expanding life beyond menopausal transition. Envision how fully embodying empowered wise woman can transform health practices, relationships, contributions, embodiment, purpose and more.

On paper vividly illustrate how you want to feel physically, emotionally, spiritually 5-10 years ahead. Sketch mindsets, community connections, environments, accomplishments marking your ideal lifescape. Make it robust stretching beyond comfort zones. This allows reverse engineering daily actions aligned with trajectories towards boldest visions not playing smallest acceptable games.

Be specific yet positive describing long term wellness, loving relationships, purposeful pursuits and provision so you recognize arrival once manifested through daily progress compounding over years.

Defining Needs & Setting Goals

With clarified vision of the vital thriving woman you're becoming fueling motivation, next define specific wellness goals improving energy, outlook and physiology through menopausal transition.

Set S.M.A.R.T. goals: Specific, Measurable, Achievable, Relevant, Time-bound. Examples:

Wellness Goals

- By December 20XX I will stabilize sleep averaging 8 hours most nights

- Within 6 months I intend feeling zero hot flash or night sweat episodes

- Over next 90 days I plan reducing average daily stress scales 20% through meditation, massage, saying no etc

Fitness Goals

- By summer 20XX I commit establishing consistent 4x weekly strength training habit

- I will add 30 minutes daily average steps by taking walks with friends

- I aim reducing body fat 3% by April through nutrition strategies

Relationship Goals

- My partner and I will schedule weekly date nights within a month

- I will initiate sex 2 times monthly to improve intimacy

- We will vacation alone by end of year reconnect adventuring

Passion Goals

- By 20XX I will clarify my purpose then publicize through defined projects

- This year I will complete informal trainings to gain skills enabling dreams

- I give myself full permission following long denied callings without guilt

Financial Goals

- Within current year max out all eligible retirement contributions

- By 20XX diversify income streams generating $XXX monthly passive revenue

- We will finalize estate planning docs to secure future legacy wishes

Draft actionable milestones across all domains longing elevation then chunk further into daily practices incrementally achieving them. Baby steps accumulate. Savour the sometimes uncomfortable growth.

Tracking Metrics that Motivate

With envisioned future secured and incremental measures defined believing progress possible, develop tracking systems quantifying efforts day-to-day. Start collecting metrics establishing baseline performance as reference progressing from.

Measure consistent inputs not just hoped for outputs since short term results depend highly factors outside your control alone.

Track items like:

- Minutes meditating, hours sleeping, steps walked, strength training sessions completed, ounces of water consumed, vegetable servings eaten etc directly fueling goals

Or document feelings consistently with scales like:

- Energy levels 1-10

- Stress/Ease levels 1-10

- Partner connection quality 1-10

- Body confidence 1-10

Technology assists easily capturing trends over time without tedious logging like apps tracking resting heart rate correlating changing exercise capacity or cycle trackers quantifying menstrual irregularities.

Pick measures that incentivize sticking with new habits through spontaneous rewards and celebration. We often estimate progress based on weight scales alone, despite weight fluctuating daily unrelated actual fat balancing muscle gained etc. Choose metrics illustrating fuller pictures that better motivate!

Rewriting Limiting Belief Stories

Beyond tangible tracking, arguably the most powerful habit established developing growth mindset involves rewriting inner belief narratives stripped of limiting assumptions, rigid identities and disempowering cultural messaging carrying unconsciously.

Our minds cling tightly to familiar old stories self-sabotaging happiness through assumptions like these needing exploration:

- I'm too old changing life narrative or physically capable pursuing goals

- It's vain/selfish prioritizing my wants after years self-sacrificing

- Real women don't openly enjoy sex after menopause

- Slowing metabolism is irreversible so why try better eating strategies

- I should feel grateful not complaining experiencing normal aging

- Reclaiming adventurous spirit means abandoning my family

Comb through mental messaging seeking distorted perceptions now outgrowing helpfulness. Does commentary align with actual circumstances or harshly judge evolving scenarios through unrealistic lenses? Beware blanket extremes, false dichotomies of good/bad thinking and fatalistic words like "always" or "never" obscuring nuance.

Actively shift self-talk celebrating growth and wins while allowing imperfection. Write fresh pages scripting more expansive empowering identities and choices catalogue every mini win boosting confidence slowly transforming belief narratives the longer you stay consistent putting in work.

Accountability Hacks

Additionally combat inertia or isolation by designing external accountability systems into goals tracking like **community**, **coaches** and **cheerleaders**. Ask trusted friends or professionals mentoring same journeys holding you kindly accountable through regular check- ins.

Enlist workout partners, nutrition accountability buddies, or mastermind groups aligned to goals. Check ego receiving guidance those ahead on paths clearing trail or who walked already before you. Follow formulas functioning for likeminded souls tweaking for unique needs.

And lastly be your own best encourager. Perfectionism proves enemy of good here with arbitrary timelines or expectations sabotaging sustainable progress rooted releasing judgment. Review efforts consistently through self-compassion lens taking pride doing your best within given circumstances showing up again, then again without harsh self-criticism certain days feel clunky.

Progress over perfection allows change taking hold long run. You've got this!

Celebrating Mini Wins

Finally infuse journey joy by intentionally celebrating mini wins and milestones frequently with rewards along the path, not just mega achievements reaching end. Enjoy the masterpiece unveiling through managing small brushstroke disciplines over years not just cheering wildly once complete final opus unveiled.

Revel in initial hot flash free days. Toast lifting new personal records at the gym. Buy flowers displaying visible progress. Savor extra rest treats between long term habits formed effortlessly. Have dance parties when bank accounts inch upwards. Watch sunsets after difficult conversations. Count blessings realizing how far you've come.

Gratitude fuels motivation realizing efforts accumulate gradually then suddenly you think "Wow journeying beyond menopause transition connected me deeply appreciating this body allows purpose and passions I never dared dreaming. I love this vital woman I'm still continuously becoming!"

That's your cue heartily cheering onward inspired for whatever next chapter adventures await! Time to call your first play.

Goal-Setting Worksheets

Let's take inspired visioning and tactical planning to next level actively listing goals across domains wanting elevation through this season plus quarterly benchmarks measuring progress. Having targets and timelines tangible engrains accountability rising to occasions.

Below find goal setting worksheets identifying health priorities, relationship growth edges, passion projects beginning, tactical financial steps securing future and whatever uniquely speaks goals wise to your circumstances. Print extra copies continuing process annually.

Be thoughtful yet comprehensive identifying growth opportunities across life domains. Also, challenge surface level wishes probing deeper perhaps values misalignment, complacency, fears or assumptions require addressing before tangible changes are possible. Discomfort signals you're stretching appropriately point of need.

Now boldly complete your blanks then revisit/revise efforts consistently reviewing if strategies effective achieving targets or require adjustments. Give grace when inevitable hiccups occur. Chunk further anything feeling overwhelming into smaller incremental action steps built sequentially towards bigger visions not demanding 100% perfection attacking everything immediately forever. You've got bandwidth pacing efforts marathon style. Let's start listing!

Health & Vitality Goals

By _______(date) I intend achieving ___(specific/measurable goal ie. normalizing sleep, stabilizing weight, reducing hot flashes, etc)

Tactical Daily Practices Supporting Goals:

____

____

____

Quarterly Benchmarks Demonstrating Progress:

____

____

____

Fitness Goals

*By _(date) I commit establishing
habit ___(specific/measurable goal ie. strength training
2x/weekly, consistent 7000 daily steps, etc)*

Tactical Daily Practices Supporting Goals:

____

____

____

Quarterly Benchmarks Demonstrating Progress:

____

____

____

Relationship Growth Goals

*By _(date) I will improve my relationship
by ___(specific/measurable goal ie. scheduling weekly date
nights, better communicating needs, addressing disconnects,
seeking counseling, etc)*

Tactical Daily Practices Supporting Goals:

____

____

____

Quarterly Benchmarks Demonstrating Progress:

____

____

____

Passion Project Goals

By _________ (date) I commit taking
step _____________ (specific/measurable goal ie. launching
blog, applying to jobs, enrolling learning programs,
beginning volunteer work, etc) towards purpose/passions

Tactical Daily Practices Supporting Goals:

____

____

____

Quarterly Benchmarks Demonstrating Progress:

____

____

____

Financial Goals

By ___________ (date) I will achieve money
milestone _________ (specific/measurable goal ie.
establishing estate planning documents, maximizing
retirement contributions, generating $XXX side income
monthly etc)

Tactical Daily Practices Supporting Goals:

____

____

____

Quarterly Benchmarks Demonstrating Progress:

____

____

____

Additional Domain Goals

By _______ (date) I intend improving _______ (relationships, personal growth, environments etc) by specifically___)

Tactical Daily Practices Supporting Goals:

____

____

____

Quarterly Benchmarks Demonstrating Progress:

____

____

____

Consistency compounds achieving envisioned goals across months and years ahead. But first begins committing dreams to paper holding self accountable. Develop vision, define measures then boldly take action! You've charted destination now pave path..

Tracking Your Progress

With inspiring big picture visions defined and incremental benchmarks queued up driving progress across spheres like health, relationships and purpose, let's ensure you implement effective tracking systems quantifying efforts and troubleshooting obstacles inevitable along journeys ahead.

Consistent measurement allows celebrating growth while also course correcting strategies if metrics indicate approaches not moving needles as hoped over time. Without data you miss the forest for the trees while patience drains feeling lacking visible payoffs perpetuating failure stories. Progress tracking brings sunshine even on stuck days.

I encourage mixing subjective data like energy or life satisfaction surveys with tangible figures like steps walked, weights lifted or dollars saved etc directly fueling goals. Apps assist capturing trends over time without tedious logging. Review measures monthly assessing what propels or impedes then tweak strategies accordingly keeping eyes the prize long term.

Here are some suggested tracking templates helping optimize efforts:

Energy & Outlook Tracking

Weekly check in scales with "1" being low and "10" being high:

- __ Energy Levels 1-10

- __ Motivation Levels 1-10

- __ Life Satisfaction 1-10

- __ Body Confidence 1-10

- __ Relationship Happiness 1-10

Identify patterns. What lifestyle factors or thought habits correlate draining or boosting your scores? How might you better support keeping outlook, self image and vitality higher avoiding dips?

Health Indicators

Log symptoms exploring potential triggers:

- Hot Flash or Night Sweat episodes

- Scale sleep hours nightly

- Record menstrual cycle details

- Stress or emotional triggers

Identify influences provoking unwelcome symptoms like sleep deficits, diet, alcohol, stress levels etc. Then experiment reducing known triggers taking control back!

Fitness Tracking

- Strength Training Sessions Completed (/4 weekly goal)

- Cardio Minutes Logged (/150 goal)

- Step Counts Averaged

- Body Measurements - scale weight, body fat %, photos etc

Progress fitness benchmarks gradually. More data better informs training adaptations needed achieving goals long run.

Relationship Efforts

- Weekly Date Nights (yes/no)

- Difficult Dialogues Completed (/# talks)

- Intimacy Encounters (sex/sensual touch sessions)

- Shared Novel Experiences (adventures/trying new things)

No need tracking every detail but high level assessments ensure you actively nurture intimacy. Measures attract focus repeated.

Financial Metrics

- Retirement Account Contributions

- % Money Allocated Towards Needs vs Wants Spending

- $ Generated From Passive Income Streams

Benchmark budget goals ensuring money redirects values like funding passions vs lifestyle inflation in areas lacking fulfillment.

Passion Project Milestones

- Completed Learning Steps (books read, trainings finished)

- Output Measures (blogs/videos created, volunteer hours logged)

- Income Generated

Whether monetizing passions now or not, track efforts to illuminate progress over time building body of work.

Journaling Insights

Beyond statistics also regularly free flow journal connections noticed from experiments implemented. Maybe certain diet upgrades energized afternoon slumps or self care rituals reduced reactivity. Note revelations, ahas! and breakthroughs too.

The key to progress lies getting comfortable assessing efforts honestly adjusting approaches not initially optimal. With supportive tracking systems built overseeing the forest for trees, breakthroughs blooms! Just begin and course correct..

Troubleshooting Setbacks

When optimizing health or consciously redirecting lifestyle trajectories, setbacks inevitably arise - motivation wanes, old habits creep back, progress plateau or unexpected circumstances throw chaos stunting forward momentum. Expect this!

But rather than harping limitations or enumerating excuses rationalizing backslides, I encourage gently troubleshooting root causes while also surrendering attachment to perfect linear ascension rates. Growth depends on missteps and course corrections. With compassionate resilience you build momentum overcoming inertia again.

This chapter offers practical troubleshooting advice getting unstuck plus inspiration celebrating revived efforts after stumbles rather than compounding failures through self-criticism. We cover:

- Reframing "Failures"

- Reigniting Lost Motivation

- When Progress Plateau

- Navigating Unexpected Circumstances

Maintain faith through wobbly phases. Consistency eventually trumps intensity when building life altering habits and visions. Now let's bust beyond barriers!

Reframing "Failures"

First mentally reframe lapses objectively as learnings rather than damning indictments of unworthiness somehow lacking willpower, capability or deserving better conditions. Setbacks indicate areas needing attention, not character flaws existentially dooming further efforts futile.

Ask curiosity questions like:

"What specifically (if anything) did this situation reveal needing to improve about my approach, expectations or environment to better support goals?"

"How can I course correct with self-compassion?"

Responsibly acknowledging causal factors allows pivoting positively. But listing limitations alone without envisioning agency to influence change further disempowers. Mentally stop catastrophic thinking predicting one "failure" surely ruining all future chances irreversibly.

Sure blindly repeating the same strategies expecting different results insanity. But setbacks naturally part of progression especially undertaking significant lifestyle shifts or consciousness expansions. Trust your resilience growing stronger through stumbles.

Reigniting Lost Motivation

When inspiration fueling new practices wanes, proactively reignite intrinsic motivations through reconnecting *why* efforts matter and what deepest desires goals aim fulfilling beyond surface aims.

Ask soul searching questions like:

"How specifically will these habit/mindset shifts improve my daily lived experience emotionally, relationally, physically, spiritually when actualized?"

"What parts of this vision still resonate with my core values and identity even when discipline lacks?"

Then list those reasons prominently somewhere visible reminding you what sparks passion on days when cultivating better habits feels tedious. Share "why" stories also with supportive friends or coaches holding you accountable reigniting inspiration.

Also scrutinize if current strategies still optimally serve evolving needs or require modifications to better aligning efforts through phases ahead with updated lifestyle contexts. Reprogress begins envisioning possibilities again.

When Progress Plateau

Assuming proper tracking metrics established quantifying efforts, first acknowledge plateaus still indicate successes maintaining new levels committing practices without backsliding. Congratulate holding standards reached thus far!

But hunger healthy progressing further. If metrics stall after consecutive months fully implementing strategies as initially prescribed, probe what changes might inject renewed results like:

- Recovering motivation above

- Seeking outside guidance from experts assessing efforts

- Changing tactics slightly surprising the body

- Boosting accountability measures

- Identifying unnecessary saboteurs remaining

Again progress rarely linear. Expect flux along the overall upward trajectory towards goals in long run. Be selectively impatient some areas and radically patient others. Balance science backed best practices with listening your body's unique rhythms and constraints this season faithfully showing up doing your best within current circumstances.

Navigating Unexpected Circumstances

When sudden unwelcome circumstances like injuries, sickness, family crises, financial disruptions etc impact lifestyle routines or emotional foundations upholding recent progress, cut self-ample slack first and foremost! Crisis management trumps everything until stabilizing fallout.

Temporarily surrender unrealistic expectations until dust settles establishing "good enough" minimum viable habits simply maintaining forward momentum awaiting relief. For example:

- Reduce exercise levels/intensities if sick or injured healing but keep moving lightly to maintain consistency forming neurological habits cemented over time

- Practice abbreviated stress management rituals if unable lengthy sessions

- Indulge comfort foods if appetite/digestion off kilter during medication treatments but consciously add greens/nutrients ensuring balanced meals again soon as possible

- Pivot intimacy encounters if menstruation arrives unexpectedly amidst perimenopause irregularity etc

Cultivating self-compassion and belief "this too shall pass" carries through brief setbacks without compounding difficulties or emotional overwhelm sabotaging recovery down the line. Hardship stretches capacity. You've got this!

Then once back solid ground, pick goals effortlessly again or reevaluate slightly realigned. Unexpected new directions sometimes get discovered only through disruptive events forcing innovation. Trust timing..

No one reaches goals optimally steadily without flux, failures or needing reimagine routes just ahead. But with consistent compassionate troubleshooting, accountability measures set supporting you and belief in own resilience, transformation sustains long run! Now reset sights boldly on horizons again after stumbles. Consistency awaits your return..

Conclusion

We've covered immense ground together exploring everything from menopausal physiology, symptom relief hacks and fitness strategies to relationship tools, financial planning, purpose alignment and more. My intention through these pages involved equipping you to leverage midlife changes forging expanded wellbeing, fulfillment and vibrant impact.

I hope you walk away from this book feeling educated, empowered and excited rising to the occasion owning your health and choices while constructing days overflowing meaning, connection and joy regardless of lifetime mile markers. Define aging on your terms!

While I can provide knowledge and suggestions, you remain pilot navigating reproductive transition and beyond through courageously embodying the leader, lover, creator, explorer, catalyst and healer already inside. Consider these words merely co-captaining your awakened wise woman spirit now ready spreading wings.

Remember progress unfolds gradually then suddenly through consistent practice. What daily disciplines and mindset shifts transform this menopausal gateway into springboard towards your greatest unfolding? How will you walk the path with more lightness and compassion for all the growth ahead?

I can't wait to witness the radical aliveness, creativity and soul purpose flowing through your days decades forward from here! Thank you for allowing me share a leg of your journey in community. Now soar unleashing the vibrant visionary within!

I wish you tremendous success optimizing vitality and purpose through the menopausal gateway and glorious years decades beyond. This exciting new era brimming expanded impact awaits your empowered leadership. Now boldly claim it!

In sisterhood and health,

Omolola Habib